BANTING SUCKS!

BANTING SUCKS!

THE **REAL** SECRET TO GENUINE WEIGHT LOSS
[WHAT LOW-CARB & BANTING FORGOT]

DR HOWARD RYBKO

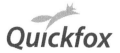

Quickfox

For my precious wife Gail and the lights of our lives
Caitlin, Paige and Gabriel

Magnificently orchestrated, groomed and edited by
Georgina Hatch.

Special thanks to Vanessa Wilson a publisher in a million,
who saved me from myself.

Thanks also to Dr Jason Fung whose insights on Type 2 diabetes
helped me to reconcile the relationship between low-carb and
weight loss that has spoiled my sleep over the past few years.

Quickfox Publishing
PO Box 494 Howard Place 7450
Cape Town, South Africa
info@quickfox.co.za
www.quickfox.co.za

First edition 2016

**BANTING SUCKS! The real secret to genuine weight loss
[what low-carb and Banting forgot]**

ISBN 10: 1533062080
ISBN 13: 9781533062086

Edited by Georgina Hatch
Cover and book design by Vanessa Wilson
Proofreading by Kelly-May Macdonald

CONTENTS

INTRODUCTION

Put down the CARBS and no one gets HURT!
Banting info on Pinterest

South Africa is Banting country; many people have 'put down the carbs'. There are Banting websites; Banting restaurants; Banting recipe books; and Banting Nazis who carb-check other people's plates at braais and family gatherings. South Africans have found their dieting Messiah and they sing its praises in business meetings, swap notes about it on social media and talk about it in Parliament.

There is even a novel about Banting, called *Death by Carbs* (Paige Nick, N&B) where The Prof who started it all is murdered in the first chapter, to the intense joy of the Health Professionals' Gang (who are suing him in real life).

Which is great, except that Banting is broken and only works sometimes for some people.

Banting is a hundred-year-old philosophy grappling with a complex modern problem. It has enough failings to suck on a grand scale.

- Banting often doesn't work for women over the age of 40

- Weight loss plateaus affect more than 90% of all long-term Banters

- Banting demonises carbs and needlessly bans many healthy food choices

- Banting treats overweight as a dietary problem when it is in fact a hormonal imbalance

- Many Banters pile on the protein, which in excess can act as kindling for cancer

- Banting targets carbs because they stimulate insulin but is totally unaware that animal protein and some dairy products are bigger culprits

- Banting does not properly address insulin resistance

These omissions have crucial health implications, which are addressed by the evolved version of Banting explained in this book.

Read this book; it will show you how to keep the good part of Banting, avoid the bad, and teach you the alterations you need to make to achieve your goal weight and maintain your health over the long term.

CHAPTER 1

A CIRCUS OF EXPERTS

'A professor is someone who talks in someone else's sleep.'
W.H. Auden

People have been Banting for the longest time

There is nothing new about the Banting concept. It was old when Robert Atkins slipped and died on an icy pavement. It was even around when the tubby undertaker William Banting had to slide downstairs backwards because he was so fat.

Believe it or not, Banting existed before William Banting was born. It just didn't have a name yet.

The French Revolution

The term Banting is used to loosely describe a low-carbohydrate eating style initially conceived by French gastronome, Jean Anthelme Brillat-Savarin, the true 'father' of Banting. He served on the National Assembly at the start of the French Revolution in 1789 and later wrote a famous book on food, in which he identified sugar and flour as the causes of obesity. His book, *Physiologie du Goût* (The Physiology of Taste) is still in print today, almost 200 years later.

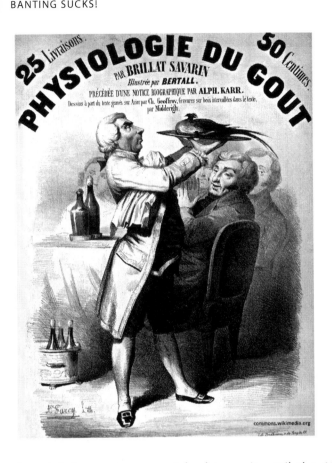

Brillat-Savarin's low-carb concept had to wait until the 1860s to become popular, sparked by Banting's distribution of over 60,000 copies of his Letter on Corpulence (published, 1863). Banting published this pamphlet, written as an open letter, telling of his struggles to lose weight and his eventual success using a diet that avoided sugar and starch. The diet became so popular that the word 'Bant' became a standard word for dieting in many countries.

'It was probably my misfortune, never to have heard of a celebrated work, La Physiologie du Goût, *by Brillat Savarin'*

William Banting

Banting, schmanting, it's all low-carb

The Banting concept is loosely connected to many variations of low carbohydrate diets such as Paleo, Atkins, Dukan and LCHF (Low-Carb-High-Fat). While they all eschew sugar and processed carbohydrates, they differ in their individual acceptance or non-acceptance of high-fat, high-protein, certain fruits and dairy products. Some of the variants like Paleo are even further divided into Lacto Paleo (dairy products allowed), Low Carb Paleo (no honey and fruits allowed) and Vegetarian Paleo (no animal-based foods).

Even Banting got Banting wrong

As soon as Banting became popular, it started to attract criticism. Its most vocal critic was Dr Wilhelm Ebstein, a well-respected German physician. Ebstein's clinical experience led him to believe that although Banting was on the right track, it allowed for too much protein to be truly healthy. (He was onto something, but more about protein later!) Ebstein's version replaced much of the protein with fat, with an emphasis on the eating of pure butter. His patients found that the extra fat reduced their hunger and their weight at the same time.

A circus of experts

Imagine a circus act, performed by the finest nutrition experts and dietitians, each one trying to convince you, the audience, that their particular diet is the best for you. Just like politicians in a TV debate, they will lie, perform circus tricks, obfuscate and twist the facts. When questioned, they become as slippery as a bar of soap in a bath.

Look! The one in the clown suit guarantees that you will lose 10 kilos in a month or your money back. See the lady in the Uncle Sam stars and stripes suit! She says you must avoid all fat because fat kills; just buy the pills she is selling on her website and in a few weeks, you will look like a swimsuit model. Wait, there's one wearing a Tim Noakes mask! He says you must eat more fat so that you can live longer and look more like him. And when you do, you won't have to worry about your high cholesterol, because no matter how much your doctor panics, cholesterol doesn't count because the higher it gets, the better it is for you; after all, it's just a money-making conspiracy by the drug companies.

What's a person to do?

It's a confusing mess when the real experts, the professors, scientists and doctors can't agree. For every professor who tells you to eat fat, another tells you fat kills. For every heart specialist who advises margarine there are two more who urge you to eat butter instead. Some doctors advise that meat is bad for you and tell you to eat poisonous soy instead. Others say eat more fruit, while their colleagues advise that fruit is too sweet and the fructose it contains will give you a fatty liver. I watched a leading nutritionist on TV the other day, sternly advising the nation to convert to vegetarianism, even as her belly bulged against the suit she was wearing. Then there's my Paleo G.P. pal in the gym who tells me that eating meat three times a day will change my life.

Then it's fish and then it's fowl and all in all, who actually knows? We are at sea, tossed in different directions by currents of deeply felt, conflicting advice.

Professor Noakes is a standout example. No one can doubt his sincerity or his good intentions. Yet 10 years ago, his lecture on carbo-loading had me advising my cyclists to stuff themselves with muesli and sweet sports drinks for days before events. Then not long ago, I sat through another of his lectures where he advised us to 'tear out the chapter on carbs' in his book, *The Lore of Running* (Human Kinetics). He was now advising us to eat fats instead of carbs (something I heartily agree with, by the way) and he then suggested I train my cyclists to ride on water and snack on macadamia nuts and biltong!

And to make it worse it seems that…

Any diet works

As a pure weight loss tool, just about any diet will work for a time.

Junk food works: Are you up for a pure junk food diet? Mark Haub, a Professor of Human Nutrition at Kansas State University certainly was. He lived on a diet of donuts, Doritos, Oreos and other junk food for 10 weeks, while trying to prove that it's not what you eat but how much of it you eat that makes you fat. It worked for him! He lost about 12 kilograms, supposedly because he ensured that his calorie intake was less than his calorie requirements.

McDonalds works: Not to be outdone, a science teacher called John Cisna dropped 16 kilograms on a pure McDonald's diet. He too kept his calorie intake below 2,000 calories a day, while subsisting on a pure McDonald's diet of Big Macs and ice cream sundaes.

These smart people believe that weight loss is about calories in, versus calories out, which certainly worked for them. But confusingly, the opposite tactic can also work...

Unlimited fat works: In 2009, Dave Asprey, the originator of the Bullet Proof Coffee recipe, set out to prove the opposite. He tried to show that you could eat a lot, do no exercise and still lose weight. His diet consisted of 70% fat with no processed sugars, which added an extra 1,500 calories to his previous daily average of 3,000. This provided him with almost double the daily intake of John Cisna, the McDonald's guy. How is it possible to explain why, instead of putting on weight from eating too much, he steadily lost weight and ended up with a six-pack for the first time in his life? Dave claims that he kept this up for almost two years and only stopped because eating so much every day became too hard to sustain indefinitely.

Grab your umbrella – confusion rains!

When faced with these kinds of contradictions, how can anyone blame the average Joe or Jane when they decide to choose a diet or lifestyle based on a magazine headline, some arbitrary personal preference, family ties, the personality of the presenter or a simple financial incentive?

How can you blame anyone who just picks a diet and hopes for the best?

CHAPTER 2

WHY BANTING IS BROKEN

'... to ascertain not only the advantages of the system now called 'Banting' but also any possible mischief in its application.'

William Banting (May 1869)

Close but no cigar

During the late 1950s, China struggled to feed its massive population and Chairman Mao began looking for ways to grow more food. He decided that China's sparrows were a problem because they ate so many grain seeds before they'd had a chance to grow. His solution was to get rid of all the sparrows in China.

Thus was born the Great Sparrow Campaign. It was enthusiastically adopted by Mao's people who set about destroying sparrow nests, smashing their eggs, killing their nestlings and shooting them out the sky. Some even resorted to banging drums and making loud noises in order to prevent flying sparrows from landing, forcing them to fly until they fell dead from the sky.

In three years, all the sparrows were gone from China.

So too were 30 million Chinese, starved to death in the resulting Great Chinese Famine, which was partly caused by massive locust swarms that gobbled up the crops. By the time Mao realised that sparrows ate locusts as well as grain, it was too late.

Mao's understanding of how the sparrows fitted into China's ecosystem was incomplete; getting rid of the sparrows was the wrong answer.

Banting is wrong about carbs

Banting's solution is to get rid of the carbs, which is also the wrong answer.

Banting's understanding of digestion and the conversion of food into energy was a great step forward – 100 years ago – but it is now time for a new way of thinking. Singling out carbs as a bad nutrient group provides too simple an answer to a complex problem and, despite working reasonably well for some, it is not a solution that works for everyone.

Banting tries to fix a hormonal imbalance by imposing a nutritional imbalance.

It's like fixing a rattle in your car's dashboard by pressing on it close to where the rattle is coming from. As soon as you let go, the rattle comes back. This leaves you with an uncomfortable solution to your rattle that forces you to steer with one hand.

In addition to its uncomfortable carb fixation, Banting has another major flaw; it presents a one-dimensional solution to a multi-dimensional problem.

In the Banting view, you are but a mouth and an anus, joined by some digestive piping. This kind of thinking pays your stressful work and personal life no heed. It also says nothing about how you should move and interact with the physical environment around you. In Banting terms, as long as you avoid carbs, all will be well.

You are a complex entity and your health encompasses much more than an arbitrary daily carb count or a series of carb avoidance strategies. Staying healthy is much more complicated than that. Soon, I will show you how to dispense with carb obsessions and how you can eat a much wider range of food.

At the same time, I will show you how Banting can be extended to cover two crucial areas: **mind and movement** in a way that will decisively transform your health and change your life without forcing you to take a course in personal training or read your way through the Internet.

But first, let's look at what's wrong with the Banting take on carbs.

Banting is about blood sugar

The foundation of Modern Banting is glucose management and the effect it has on insulin levels. It mistakenly singles out carbohydrates as the only food group that spikes insulin and thus prescribes a reduction of carbs to keep blood sugar levels as stable as possible. This reduces insulin spikes and, as a result, prevents fat production and promotes weight loss.

Unfortunately, the Banting theory is not accurate enough. It presses on the dashboard to stop the rattle but it fails to address the real problem, which manifests in two specific instances:

- A high proportion of women over forty struggle to lose weight on Banting.
- Almost every Banter eventually hits a weight-loss plateau.

Women over forty

*'I gained some weight even though I was
doing everything right.'*
Low-carb consultant who worked with Dr Atkins for 30 years

There is a whole weight loss industry that is sustained by legions of women over forty who simply cannot lose weight. The quote above from Jackie Eberstein, a registered nurse and life-long low-carb consultant, says it all; sometimes even experienced low-carbers can't lose weight by Banting. She also says that when she trains professionals, the most common question they ask is how to deal with slow weight loss in older women. It is so widespread that it is actually a pandemic.

I recently received an email newsletter from a weight-loss expert and author of a bestselling New York Times' diet book that promises a 15-pound weight loss in three weeks. Her mail discloses that she still struggles with tight clothes and has been forced to wear 'Not Your Daughter's' jeans since she turned 45. She also admits to being recently measured at 30% body fat, which she blames partially on aging. This is shocking when you consider that many of my patients are unhappy at 25% body fat. Surely low-carb theory is missing something when even the experts can't make it work properly?

I too have had my share of failures. Take Jo-Anne for example; a 41-year-old serial dieter, who worked as a receptionist, ate badly and did no exercise. She was 20 kilograms overweight when she came to see me and, despite my best efforts, she was still 20 kilos overweight two months later when she left. It seemed so easy in the beginning. I stopped her carbs, which were in everything she ate. I upped her exercise from zero to walking twice a week. I even got her to move more at work by downloading an app on her phone, which reminded her to stand up every 30 minutes so that she did not sit for too long. Nothing worked. Her weight stubbornly remained the same until she decided that I was incapable of helping her and ditched me for a course of HCG injections, which she ordered on the internet.

Maybe Jo-Anne was cheating on me. I told myself that she was not following the diet properly and that was the reason she was unable to lose weight. Surely her lack of results could not be caused by my flawed dietary advice? For a while, the excuse of poor compliance allowed me to avoid facing the reality that my Banting B.S. only worked sometimes.

Then I met Celia the cyclist, who removed any notion I may have harboured about poor compliance as the reason for the diet's failure. Celia was 55 years old and she was so active and so disciplined that it made my muscles ache just to talk to her. She rode her bike every weekday morning from 5 am to 7 am and still trained in the gym some evenings. Over weekends she would race her bike; once she rode 200 kilometres a day for three days just to get to an event. Still, Celia carried seven extra kilograms around her middle that would not budge.

Initially, I was sure that I could help her because she would be a model patient and would carry out my every suggestion to the letter. Yet despite her following an extreme low-carb diet combined with extreme exercise, she did not lose a single kilogram over six rigorous weeks.

Thus it became clear to me that it wasn't the application of Banting low-carb theory that was at fault; the theory itself was to blame.

Weight loss plateaus

Almost everyone who goes Banting eventually reaches a plateau, at which point fat loss stalls and some weight remains. Many find that despite initial good results, they end up retaining some stubborn belly fat that just won't go away. This effect seems to become worse with age.

The question is why does this happen?

Surely if the Banting principle is correct, then these weight loss plateaus should happen far less often. People who Bant properly for long enough should become lean, but few do.

While it is possible for some determined Banters to find their way past this point, most fail. Those who succeed often do so by employing extreme measures such as even greater carb restriction or a combination of restricted calorie intake and intense exercise. Many of the patients who come to me seeking advice are disciplined enough to have tried both these methods but still cannot achieve their desired weight loss.

Plateaus are big money spinners for weight loss practitioners. Many diet specialists claim to have methods that are 'guaranteed' to work and irrespective of their results, they never seem to be short of customers.

The Doc's spare tyre

When it comes to plateaus, I am a good example. I adopted a low-carb (Banting) lifestyle in 2012 and quickly experienced a weight loss of 10% of my original body mass. Over the next three years, I followed a strict low-carb diet, never consuming more than 25 grams of carbs a day. I also exercised intensely, working out five or six times a week; yet despite this regime, a few kilos of stubborn belly fat remained.

Sure, the spare tyre was small enough to hide or explain away as 'old age' but it still irked me. Just as it had done for most of my patients, low-carb solved most of my weight problem but still did not return a completely satisfactory result. This was especially true on a medical level because my waking blood sugar levels hovered stubbornly at the upper limits of normal.

I struggled with this problem for months, obsessively trying to understand how it was possible to have almost diabetic blood sugars when I was not eating any sugar. It took me a long time to finally accept that it was Banting that was flawed and not my application of it.

Which gets us to the point…

Why does the Banting take on digestion suck?

It sucks because it targets blood sugar levels and singles carbs out as the sole culprit, which is simply not good enough.

Banting holds that the consumption of high-carbohydrate processed foods results in weight gain in most, but not all, people. This is equivalent to Mao's observation that crop yields are reduced because the swallows eat grain seeds. Both assumptions mirror reality closely enough to be useful in certain circumstances; however, neither assumption is correct.

William Banting's 'high starch intake makes you fat' observation has been vindicated by medical research as well as a multitude of treatment successes stretching from the 1860s to modern times. On top of this, medical science has proved countless times that the consumption of high-carbohydrate processed foods spike blood sugar levels, which then spike insulin levels and lead to the inevitable accumulation of body fat. The main suspect has always been sugar and the lens through which we look has always been the level of sugar in the blood.

Blood sugar levels are easy and inexpensive to monitor and all diabetic treatments are primarily based on lowering these levels.

While it is indisputable that high blood sugar levels are unhealthy, what if we have been victims of a classic Hollywood misdirection? What if we have been duped into focusing all our attention on the obvious suspect and, because we have achieved some success with this reasoning, we have allowed the real murderer to escape?

The usual suspects

Have you ever watched the most famous misdirection movie of all time? 'The Usual Suspects' tells the tale of an enigmatic psychopath called Keyser Soze, seen through the eyes of Verbal, a pathetic cripple who is one of Soze's victims. As the movie unfolds, we are introduced to a variety of likely suspects, but the one character we never suspect is the weakling Verbal. At the end of the movie, as Verbal is released from custody, he drops his cripple pose, lights a cigarette and strides purposefully toward the black luxury sedan that has arrived to fetch him. A voice in the background says 'The greatest trick the devil ever pulled was convincing the world he didn't exist'.

In recent years, we have always regarded fat and sugar as the usual suspects. Many clues point to them, but what if they are just red herrings and the real killer is hidden in plain view?

What if we are so blasé about the real killer that our doctors dole it out by the bucketful, ordering dose increases over the phone or tossing casual prescriptions across their desks? What if we are so hoodwinked by the killer's innocence that most doctors don't even measure its levels during routine check-ups?

What if some experts are so comfortable with its safety that they add it to the drips of diabetic patients who are being treated in ICU after suffering a heart attack? Who would suspect that by doing this they virtually guarantee the future death by heart attack of every second patient treated with it?

What if the real devil is insulin?

Let's take a quick look at our real enemy.

CHAPTER 3

KNOW YOUR ENEMY: ITS NAME IS INSULIN

'My doctor said insulin occurs naturally in our bodies and cannot harm us.'

Internet post

In early 1921, two research assistants at Toronto University nonchalantly spun a coin to decide which one of them would work on a new diabetes research project. Had they known that the winner would receive the Nobel Prize for Medicine, they would surely have taken their coin toss a tad more seriously.

Charlie Rose won the toss and the privilege to work with the small town Canadian doctor he had just been introduced to. The doctor's name was Fredrick Banting, no relation to our Mr William Banting, and he was trying to isolate a mysterious substance believed to be made in the pancreas; a mystery substance that was somehow connected to the high blood sugars that killed most diabetics in those times. Banting's goal was to perfect an experimental operation on dogs that no one had yet been able to successfully carry out. He succeeded and in the process saved many lives. After winning the Nobel for this work, he donated his patent for insulin to Eli Lilly Corporation for a token $1. Sadly, Banting's generosity did nothing to shield him from misfortune; he was killed in World War II when the air-force bomber he was flying in crashed into a harbour in Newfoundland.

Eli Lilly did a lot better. Less than two years after starting insulin production, they had sold over 50 million units and founded a billion dollar industry in the process.

Insulin economics 101

> *'Human insulin market worth $42 billion by 2019'*
>
> *marketsandmarkets.com*

Initially, insulin was cheap to manufacture and cheap to buy. However, the inexorable laws of economics came into play and a highly competitive insulin industry quickly developed. Selling gallons of insulin became big business and an army of sales reps was marshalled to pressurise doctors into prescribing more and more of the stuff. Fuelled by the pumping of human greed glands, insulin prices have increased by over 300% in the last 10 years alone.

One does not need the deductive powers of Sherlock Holmes to work out why doctors are under pressure to get patients onto insulin as soon as possible. There is little resistance to this pressure because most doctors believe insulin to be harmless and, as a result, they prescribe it in ever-increasing doses to a seemingly limitless market of diabetic customers.

What is insulin?

Insulin is an anabolic hormone made in the pancreas. It is produced by almost all animals and has been around for over a billion years. Insulin is intimately involved with growth. It drives sugars into the cells, the storage of excess energy as fat and, in the right conditions, it grows muscle. Insulin attaches itself to cell walls, opening a doorway for glucose and other nutrients to move out of the blood and into the cells. This movement of glucose into the cells lowers the level of sugar in the blood.

Because it is strongly anabolic, insulin is used by some body-builders to preserve the muscle mass they gain during training. To do this, they drink supplements high in sugar and protein at the same time as they inject insulin. This increases the flow of glucose and amino acids into their muscles and enhances growth; however, it requires great care to ensure muscle growth without fat gain. It works, but some of the bodybuilders die when they inject too much insulin and slip into a diabetic coma.

The real problem is not a handful of ignorant bodybuilders. The real problem affects a much larger group of people; over half the earth's population walk around with chronically raised insulin levels.

Too much insulin is bad for you

There is little doubt that prolonged exposure to high insulin levels causes health issues. However, in many cases it is not easy to identify insulin as the cause because there are so often many other more obvious suspects. High blood pressure is a good example; while it is likely that this occurs as a result of high insulin levels, many other factors such as high dietary sodium levels and stress are often blamed.

Here is a list of some of the possible consequences of sustained high insulin levels for you to consider. Look around you and you will see many people in your daily life who are affected by one or more of these, many of which are blamed on other causes:

- Tiredness
- Weight gain
- Hunger
- High blood sugar levels
- High blood pressure
- Heart disease
- Diabetes
- Cancer
- Low thyroid function
- Depression
- Brain fog and an inability to concentrate

How can insulin be bad for us when we practically swim in it?

CHAPTER 4

DROWNING IN INSULIN

'I was astonished to encounter no cases of cancer.'
Albert Schweitzer

Early in his career, Alberto Villodo, anthropologist and psychologist, was hired by a large Swiss pharmaceutical company to journey into the deepest parts of the Amazon in an attempt to discover ancient remedies for cancer and heart disease. His employers hoped they could bring these cures back to the West, patent them and turn them into blockbuster drugs. His quest took him to jungle places so isolated from civilisation that the children living there would often rub his skin to see if the 'white dirt' would come off.

After living with these people for six months, he returned to the USA. He told his employers that he could find no ancient cures for cancer or heart disease in the Amazon because these diseases did not exist.

He was not the first.

Albert Schweitzer, doctor, explorer and Nobel Prize winner, spent most of his life in the remote African jungles of Gabon. He arrived in Lamberene in 1913 and built his hospital on a piece of land that he had wrested from the jungle. Even before his hospital was completed, his first patients started to trickle in.

They kept flowing in at a rate of 30 to 40 patients a day and more than 20 years would pass before he saw his first cancer or heart disease case. By that time, the locals had begun incorporating Western processed foods like grains and sugar into their diet.

The absence of cancer and heart disease in pre-industrial societies has been reported by other missionary or adventure-minded doctors in areas all over the globe.

All primitive societies survive on natural foods which they source from the environment around them. Irrespective of the composition of these foods, whether animal protein, vegetable or fruit, the consumption of them *in their natural state* does not sharply raise blood sugar levels.

Meal frequency in these societies is another differentiator. Most primitive societies eat larger meals at infrequent intervals. This produces higher but more infrequent insulin spikes and does not induce insulin resistance; it is highly likely that the people of these societies had low average blood insulin levels, as shown by some studies of surviving hunter-gatherer communities. Compare this to Western agricultural societies who eat processed foods and have considerably higher average insulin levels.

Is it possible that the rise of cancer and heart disease correspond to the rise of insulin levels in 'civilised' societies?

Modern insulin levels

Worldwide average insulin levels have increased as a result of two factors. Most people eat all the time and when they eat their diet normally consists of processed foods, sugars and grains. This pattern of continual grazing completely contradicts our ancestral heritage where our ancestors were not normally accustomed to a limitless food supply. They ate when they could and their genetics developed to accommodate times of feast as well as times of famine. Their systems developed to easily cope with a few days without food.

I believe that modern insulin levels are at least double the prevailing levels in ancestral times; a conclusion that is supported by many studies. For example, the findings of the 2007–2008 NHANES (National Health and Nutrition Examination Survey) study of around 40,000 people across the USA showed that people who consume processed foods have average fasting insulin levels over four times higher than those who eat high-fat diets, which do not stimulate insulin. This explains why Dave Asprey, the guy I mentioned in the chapter 'A circus of experts', could eat so much and still lose weight; the fat he ate drove his insulin levels down, resulting in weight loss.

People who are overweight or those who eat a high sugar diet often have much higher fasting insulin levels, sometimes with levels as high as double or triple accepted maxima.

Having so many people walking around with sustained high levels of a potent growth hormone in their blood will greatly increase their individual susceptibility to diseases of the heart, blood vessels and cancer.

We can be sure that both Alberto Villodo's Amazon villagers and Albert Schweitzer's Africans had low fasting insulin levels. They were also cancer and heart disease free. We, on the other hand, are not. Sustained higher average insulin levels are genetically unexpected and our bodies have no natural defense against the long-term consequences of this condition.

I know some experts will disagree with me, citing our toxic modern environment as the root cause of the high rates of these diseases. While there is no doubt that modern conditions do exert some effect, remember that Albert Schweitzer's first heart disease and cancer patients were still living in a pre-industrial jungle environment when they became ill. All they needed was a few years on sugar and grains to make them sick.

What causes chronically raised insulin levels?

Ask anyone and they will tell you that they are caused by sugar and carbs, which is only partially correct, because as you have learned by now, protein does it too.

However, the spikes caused by food are not the real problem!

The real cause is continual eating.

CHAPTER 5

INSULIN RESISTANCE — BANTING'S MAJOR WEAKNESS

*'I do moderate exercise, and I try to eat pretty well...
But hey, I'm putting on the insulin tyre like everybody else,
but that's just a function of getting older.'*
Mel Gibson – www.comingsoon.net

No stranger to making the occasional misconceived public statement, Mr Gibson does it again. Sorry Mel, but your spare tyre is not a function of getting older. It's caused by something called insulin resistance and if you call me during office hours, I will show you how to get rid of it in time for your next movie.

Before we look at what insulin resistance actually is, let's do a quick summary of what we have learned so far in Tweet-sized chunks.

Banting does not work properly because:

- It is based on stabilising blood sugar by limiting carbs
- It wrongly assumes that only carbs raise insulin levels
- It does not properly understand how insulin works; nor does it teach us how to manage insulin levels
- **Critically, it does not always normalise diabetic blood profiles, sometimes even in those who lose weight**

Insulin is the real danger to your health:

- You have to focus on reducing your insulin levels in order to lose weight and dramatically improve your long-term health profile
- Over 50% of the population walk around with chronically raised insulin levels, which is behind the explosion of heart disease and cancer in modern society
- The core of Banting's weakness lies in its failure to deal directly with insulin resistance

So what is insulin resistance?

Mel Gibson's spare tyre is a direct result of insulin resistance, which is caused by too much insulin. The question is: what is insulin resistance?

Insulin is the key to the door in the cell wall that lets glucose in. Without insulin, the door cannot open and glucose will accumulate in the blood.

Insulin resistance happens when it gets harder and harder to open the door.

Think about it as if you were opening your front door. Normally, you depress the handle and push the door which swings open easily. However, what happens when it gets windy outside and the wind pushes against the door? The extra pressure from the wind makes the door harder to open and the windier it becomes, the harder you have to push to open the door.

Insulin resistance works in a similar way. The more resistant your cells become to insulin, the harder it becomes for insulin to open the door. As it gets harder, more and more insulin has to be made to get the door to open.

Over time, as the resistance to insulin worsens, it causes two issues. Blood sugar levels start to rise as the insulin becomes less effective at keeping them down; at the same time, average insulin levels start to rise because the pancreas has to keep making more to get the job done.

Modern medicine has a lot to say about the control of blood sugar (glucose). In fact, it would not be inaccurate to say that it obsesses about blood glucose levels. Modern medicine believes that the high blood sugars in diabetes are the root cause of all its negative health consequences which include heart disease, high blood pressure and nerve damage. That insulin levels are pretty much ignored is underscored by the insouciance with which medics push diabetics to use more and more insulin.

This is a grave mistake because as we know by now, insulin is dangerous. In the long term, high insulin levels are probably more dangerous than high blood sugar levels. This is clear from the results of a number of studies that have sought to improve diabetic outcomes by closely controlling blood sugar levels with more insulin.

The ACCORD study – proof that insulin is more dangerous than high blood sugar

This 2008 study was designed to demonstrate the value of extremely tight blood sugar level control in a group of over 10,000 diabetics. For years doctors have believed that the better the glucose control in diabetic patients, the better their health will be. As a result, they teach type 2 diabetic patients to watch their blood sugar levels and to inject with as much insulin as necessary to keep blood sugar levels as low as possible.

Well, the ACCORD study proved this notion to be false. It showed that more intensive control of sugar levels leads to an unanticipated and dramatic increase in overall death rates in diabetics. So dramatic, in fact, that they stopped the trial early to reduce the risks to the lives of patients in the trial. This increase in death rates can only have resulted from greater use of insulin and insulin-enhancing agents by subjects of the trial.

What causes insulin resistance?

Eating all day.

Yes, I know that eating processed foods and drinking high sugar drinks are linked to insulin resistance, but it's quite likely that the body can cope better with these insults than is popularly believed. I think that the real devil can be found in the effects of continuous insulin stimulation.

Insulin was designed to work in bursts. It is released in response to a meal and then subsides until the next meal, which would normally come many hours later. Insulin, like all hormones, works best when released in a pulsatile manner with strong rises interspersed with periods of calm which, over time, produce a wavelike rise and fall.

However, our modern lifestyle does not allow for enough time between meals for insulin levels to subside. We are driven by our eating of processed foods, marketing machines and our medical specialists who insist that we never be hungry. Eating continually as we do pushes up insulin levels and ensures that these levels stay up all day.

Most modern people don't allow themselves to experience hunger.

We wake up and expect to eat breakfast, which has become something of a Human Right. Most doctors sternly remind their patients that 'breakfast is the most important meal of the day'. Mothers are taught that by allowing their children to go to school without breakfast, they fail in their duties. Then, after having eaten breakfast, most of us seem to look forward to our mid-morning tea break, followed by lunch, then afternoon tea and then supper, which cannot be complete without an after-dinner snack. Some people even eat again before they go to bed.

Can you imagine how this continual grazing affects our insulin levels, which don't get a chance to drop during the day? How do these sustained levels of potent anabolic hormones affect the tissues of our body? How do the insulin receptors of these tissues know how to respond to this kind of unnatural stimulation by insulin for 12 to 18 hours a day?

It seems to me that cancer and growth in the lining of blood vessels (atherosclerosis) would surely be the logical result of this kind of sustained stimulation. It makes sense that the rise of cancer and heart disease in modern society is a direct result of the sustained insulin levels most of us live with.

The road to insulin resistance

Understanding this slow process and experiencing it are altogether different. As I found out one icy evening many years ago, walking my mother, a diabetic for almost 15 years, through an icy parking lot. To her family, she appeared to be fine, a little overweight and a little sleepy at times, but still functioning well. I had watched passively over the years as her diabetologist gradually increased her meds, pushing her along the insulin resistance road. He started her off on a single pill, which increased gradually to many pills and finally to insulin injections before every meal. I meekly accepted his dictates as he applied the dogma of the day, feeding my mom, who already suffered from too much insulin, more and more insulin.

That night, the sound of footsteps rushing towards us out of the darkness froze us in our tracks. I craned backward to see a rag-covered old man close behind us, brandishing an object in his hand. 'Stop!' he said. I turned and took a step toward him, raising my hands palms out. Then, as I had been taught in self-defence classes I said, 'Please, don't hurt us.'

'No, no,' he said, waving the object in his hand in my mother's direction, 'I have her shoe.'

Incredibly, my mom's shoe had fallen off while she was walking, yet she had continued, unaware that the icy, graveled ground underfoot was drawing blood with every step. So numbed were the nerves to her legs that she could neither feel the loss of her shoe nor the sharp stones she walked on.

You don't get to be like my mom overnight. It takes years of travel along the road to insulin resistance before you hear the word 'diabetes' and your name spoken in the same sentence. I hope that it will never happen to you but if it does, don't be surprised if you shake your head and tell your doctor that it's not possible, because you feel fine.

My biggest worry about Banting

Just in case I haven't made my point clear, please bear with me and let me repeat myself: Banting plus exercise predictably leads to weight loss in most males (and in some females) but it does not always result in normalised blood sugar or insulin levels. This is because it is treating a hormonal disorder by restricting a single nutrient group. This leads to the unfortunate situation where sometimes you have a fit and healthy looking patient, with a resting heart rate below 50 and a random glucose within normal limits, BUT you still find a pre-diabetic blood profile when you dig deeper. These patients may also have borderline hypertension.

This can result in the unfortunate situation where you have Banters walking around with pre-diabetes, who look like a million dollars and behave as if they are Teflon-coated, but diabetes and the consequences of insulin resistance are still very much in play.

Diabetes, stealthy as a cat on the hunt, sneaks up on you.

CHAPTER 6

WHY YOU SHOULD FEAR DIABETES

'Every six seconds someone dies from diabetes.'
International Diabetes Federation

I remember being mildly irritated as Samuel, a 50-year-old diabetic, was allocated to me just before the end of a long night in the emergency ward at Baragwanath Hospital in Soweto. Life as a medical slave in Africa's largest hospital during the dark years of Apartheid could be a bitch. In the world of tenured medical slaves; known, irrespective of gender, as 'housemen', there could be no greater disaster than being allocated a diabetic patient just before the end of your shift.

Diabetic patients were feared because they could take hours to stabilise and needed regular blood tests to assess the progress of their treatment. In those days, you had little option but to hoof it to the lab, scribble the results down and then double back to the ward. Hard work, especially after 24 hours on your feet, as part of the only emergency station serving a city of two million people living without electricity or running water.

My irritation vanished as soon as I stepped through the curtains around Samuel's bed. He was terrified, and lay stiff and silent on the bed. His eyes, full of fear, locked onto my face as I examined him. On a chair by his side, bag perched on her tightly squeezed knees, sat his wife. Her voice trembled as she told me that they had woken well before dawn and while she was making their tea, Samuel first complained about a pain in his calf. Worried, she asked him to check his blood sugar, which turned out to be sky-high, so she gave him a shot of rapid acting insulin. Then as they sat and sipped their tea, Samuel's calf began to visibly swell. His growing pain spurred the couple to abandon their kitchen table and slip into the dark alleyways in search of an early morning taxi that was prepared to rush them to the emergency room.

As I examined him, the lower part of Simon's leg continued to swell visibly, making me realise that I was out of my depth. I called the surgical registrar I reported to for help; he had a brief look and panicked too, calling for our head of unit who kept shaking his head. Together, we rolled Samuel onto a gurney and ran the squeaking, juddering gurney to theatre, dispensing with the procedure requiring us to wait for the theatre staff to transport him.

We operated a short while later, to find an aggressive gas-forming bacteria at work. It was multiplying at a frightening rate in Samuel's sugar-sweetened tissues and we had little choice but to amputate below the knee. Samuel came round in the recovery ward at midday, silent but smiling hopefully at us as we clustered around his bed. Hoping to prevent further spread of the voracious organism, we doused him intravenously with our most potent antibiotics, using levels far in excess of the recommended dosages. To no avail. Two hours later, in desperation, we took him back to surgery, this time to amputate his leg above the knee.

Disheartened and exhausted, I went home and tried in vain to catch a few hours of sleep. I returned early the next morning and went straight to Samuel's bed in ICU. One look told me that we were losing him and I paged the chief of surgery, who arrived at a run. Less than a minute later, he turned away from the bed and headed for the door. "I'll meet you in theatre," he said.

Samuel was then subjected to a mutilating surgical procedure called a hindquarter resection. We removed the remainder of his leg and sawed off part of his bony pelvis along with all the attached muscles. Samuel survived the operation but he never regained consciousness. As night began to fall on Soweto, the rampant infection spreading through his body took him.

Here was the beast at work, unmasked in its full fury, killing in a way that is every bit as terrifying as any Hollywood murder scene.

Click to select your ending

It is predicted that Hollywood will sometime in the near future produce movies that allow viewers to select their preferred ending from a list. This will give viewers choices like: 'Click 1 for a happy ending'; 'Click 2 for a sad ending'; and so on.

Life, like the movies, has many alternate endings and when people think about ways of dying they tend to opt for bigger, more picturesque endings rather than dying like Samuel. Some of the more 'popular' endings are an airplane crash, a plunge down a lift-shaft or being eaten alive by wild animals. And for those a little short of inspiration, Hollywood or the daily TV news provides plenty of material.

Happily, your odds of dying a graphic death are remote. Being eaten alive by wild animals is the most remote at about one in 20 million, while your chances of dying in an airplane crash are around one in a million. Unlikely or not, graphic deaths like these tend to loom large in our imagination and garner far more airtime than they deserve.

We seldom think about the things that are much more likely to kill us. As Peter Sandman, international risk consultant puts it: 'The risks that kill people and the risks that upset people are completely different'.

So ask yourself: if it's risks that kill rather than fears, which risk do you think is the most likely to kill you? Perhaps you can find inspiration from the quote at the top of this chapter.

Samuel was not alone; one death every six seconds adds up to an awful lot of people. Especially when on a personal level, your chances of dying from the consequences of insulin resistance or diagnosed diabetes are less than one in four, making it a clear favourite. It affects all of us, young and old, fat or thin; excluding accidents, almost everyone living in a developed country has some form of raised insulin levels that will ultimately kill them.

Over time, raised insulin levels cause diabetes but also lead to many diseases like heart disease and cancer. Raised insulin levels are a direct result of poor diet and lifestyle choices and can be avoided or reversed with relative ease.

Which is where this book comes in.

Now that you know more about the dark side of diabetes, let me show you why you should check your blood sugar.

CHAPTER 7

WHY YOU HAVE TO CHECK YOUR BLOOD SUGAR

'The truth will set you free, but first it will piss you off.'

Unknown comedian

Meet Dr K, who's fit as a fiddle. He's a regular 'fun runner' who trains twice a week with his running group. He also goes to gym regularly and does an indoor cycling class or a circuit at his local gym.

In the past, he would cheerily acknowledge that he was a little overweight. 'I may carry a little extra around my middle,' he would say as he affectionately patted the muffin top peeping over his belt, 'but I'm stronger than Russia!'

He tried hard to follow the eating advice he doled out to his patients; reduce fats, no sugar in his coffee, eat healthy grains and fruit. He also advised his patients to eat six small meals a day to keep their weight down and their blood sugar levels under control.

Dr K considered himself to be perfectly healthy until the day when a constant stream of patients left him urgently needing to pee. Desperate, he seized a gap between patients to empty his bladder into the large medical beaker on his desk, which was how his next patient found him as she walked in unannounced.

Unzipped and unfinished, he nonchalantly waved his astonished patient to a chair, all the while desperately thinking of a way to save face. Seeing a tube of testing strips within reach, he grabbed one and casually popped it into the brimming beaker of urine. 'Sorry about that,' he said, 'It couldn't wait; I had to test my sugar.'

Later, after the patient had left, he glanced at the test strip and was shocked to see it had turned an angry purple color, indicating a strongly positive result. Sure enough, blood tests confirmed that his blood glucose was double the upper limit of normal. While it shocked him to find that he was diabetic, his biggest shock came from the realisation that he had no idea he was sick. He had been blinded by a smug belief in his physical fitness and medical knowledge.

He then embarked on a series of measures (part of this book) which, nearly five years later, continues to spare him from the heart attack that killed his father when he was of a similar age. In those days his waking blood sugar was between eight and ten (over seven and you're officially a diabetic). Today it's in the low fours! He also dropped 10 kilos in weight and stopped all his meds, including an anti-depressant that he was too proud to admit he was addicted to.

Medical professionals

Where does that leave you, when a dedicated, well-intentioned medical professional like Dr K, who, despite his training, can walk around for years with raised blood sugar?

I think that the key message here is that out-of-control blood sugar is a silent nemesis that anyone can carry.

How to check your blood sugar

It is best to start off with a fasting blood glucose test. Simply wake up one morning and, before eating or drinking anything, go and get your blood sugar measured. An easy way to do this is to find a local pharmacy that offers this service. You can also go to your doctor or to a clinic nearby.

If this initial test is anywhere near the upper limit of the normal, I strongly suggest that you get yourself a meter and start doing daily checks until you know exactly what is going on with your blood sugar.

Fasting blood glucose levels in mmol/l (8 hours after last eating)

As defined by the World Health Organization:
- 7.0 or above = Diabetes
- 6.1 to 6.9 = Impaired fasting glucose (also called pre-diabetes)
- 6.0 to 5.6 = High normal
- 5.5 or below is preferred

Testing yourself

Get yourself a blood glucose tester. These can often be sourced for free at your local pharmacy. They will often give you the meter as long as you pay for the first box of test strips, which is a really good investment. It may seem a little fiddly at first but you will soon master the art of pricking yourself!

Daily testing will enable you to gain an understanding of how different meals and snacks affect your blood sugar levels. Your key to health is controlling your insulin levels and the most practical way to do this is by monitoring actual blood sugar levels.

Don't let the minor complexities of using a glucose meter put you off. It is worth the effort to know your blood sugar levels. It's not overkill because living with out-of-control sugar and insulin levels can cost you your health.

Testing your fasting insulin level

In addition to knowing your blood sugar, I would strongly recommend that you have your fasting insulin level tested. You cannot do this at home or by pinprick; the test has to be done by a medical laboratory service. You may be able to order the test yourself or you can ask your doctor to order it for you.

If you are overweight or carry some belly fat, I would go so far as to say that taking this test is mandatory for you. Study your results carefully. Remember that high insulin levels are dangerous and be aware that the normal range tolerated by the laboratory may be somewhat too lenient at its upper limits.

If your initial fasting insulin result is high, implement some of the measures presented in this book and then re-test after eight to ten weeks. Keep testing regularly to make sure that your levels come down to low normal levels.

CHAPTER 8

EXCESS PROTEIN — BANTING'S MAJOR WEAKNESS

'Protein intake is a regulator of IGF-1, a risk factor for prostate cancer, breast cancer, colon cancer and many other cancers.'
Professor Luigi Fontana, human systems biologist

The Banting hive-mind has reached a consensus that assumes high-protein intake is good for both health and weight loss. This is wrong on both counts.

High protein intake can:

- Prevent weight loss
- Accelerate weight gain
- Promote a range of cancers

Since it has, of late, become *de rigueur* for the socially active to be seen to be 'Banting', I often become involved in conversations with Banting experts and Banting haters alike. Conversations can at times become heated, leaving me on the receiving end of sweeping statements such as this pearl from a recent business dinner: 'I don't know how people can manage this Banting; I mean, who wants to eat meat all day?'

Banting is regarded by many as a high-protein diet and people seem to think that it swaps carbs for animal-based protein. When I can, I do my best to remind them that Banting, done properly, is a high-fat diet and suggest ways for them to incorporate more fat into their diet.

Excess protein in a Banting environment

When one is Banting, there often seems to be little choice but to increase protein intake to replace the missing carbs. This also happens when preparing food using one of the many Banting recipes or when buying off-the-shelf Banting products, because they all have to substitute either protein or fat for the carbs they remove. As a result, it is easy for Banters to exceed normal daily protein intake limits.

While some scientists believe that the regular intake of too much protein is unhealthy, this has never been conclusively proved to occur in healthy individuals. I do nevertheless feel that there is some merit to this belief and caution against excessive protein intake.

From a Banting perspective, overdosing on protein causes two major problems. It slows or reverses weight loss and it raises some long-term health issues.

Banters beware

First, high protein intake can lead to an increase in sugars in the blood, the exact outcome the Banting diet set out to avoid. Excess protein is converted to sugar in a slow but steady process called gluconeogenesis and because of this, a low-carb diet can sometimes become a high-carb diet and can manifest as higher than expected blood sugar levels in carb-sensitive people.

Second, and perhaps more importantly, animal protein, specifically meat and cheese, pushes up insulin levels. In traditional Banting, these products are given the green light because they don't affect blood sugar levels but they are, in fact, fattening because of their effect on insulin levels. If you struggle to drop weight despite being careful about your carb intake, these should be your primary suspects. Consider reducing the quantities you eat rather than dropping them completely.

Beware of protein shakes: The reason that meat and cheese stimulate insulin is because they contain high levels of protein building blocks called BCAAs (Branch Chain Amino Acids). These BCAAs are found in high concentrations in whey products and often form the basis of protein shakes and muscle-building drinks. Be aware that your protein shake will kick your insulin levels and is far more likely to grow you some extra fat instead of the extra muscle it promises.

(If you are looking for a way to grow some muscle, see the section 'Growing muscle legally', which explains the use of a BCAA protein shake to hack muscle growth.)

Kidney stones

Another area where excess protein intake may cause issues is in the kidneys. The evidence confirming this is not in yet and while normal Banting kidneys may not be at risk, high protein intake is definitely not recommended for people with existing kidney problems.

Some studies have shown that high protein diets increase acid loads in the blood, which can lead to higher calcium levels in the kidneys. Having higher calcium levels in the kidneys will increase the likelihood of kidney stone formation.

Anecdotally, kidney stones are definitely an issue and many renal specialists feel that low-carb diets cause a predisposition to stone formation. Until this debate is settled conclusively, I strongly advise all Banters and low-carb dieters to ensure that they drink plenty of water, especially during hot weather and when exercising; and that they follow my advice to limit protein consumption!

Long-term ill effects

> *'...convincing evidence that a high-protein diet – particularly if the proteins are derived from animals – is nearly as bad as smoking for your health.'*
> Dr Valter Longo, Professor of longevity

Dr Longo gained international exposure in 2014 with the quote above. While he is probably being intentionally sensational, regular consumption of too much protein is almost certainly bad for your health. It will make you age quicker and increase your risk of cancer.

Many studies have revealed increased overall health risks. Part of these risks is related to the stimulatory effect that animal protein has on levels of IGF-1 (Insulin-like Growth Factor 1). IGF-1 promotes cell growth and acts in a similar way to insulin. Its growth-promoting properties are somehow linked to increased cancer risks in adults, especially breast and prostate cancer. People who are born without IGF-1 don't get cancer, although they do suffer from stunted growth.

High IGF-1 levels also make you age quicker. Studies of round-worms called C. elegans have demonstrated some startling anti-aging results. We are a long way from roundworms, but it is more than a little interesting to find that worms with low IGF-1 levels live up to 90% longer (an average of 57 days) than normal.

While there are also clear indications that low IGF-1 levels have bad effects, mainly on the heart and circulation, it would still seem prudent to be wary of eating too much animal protein.

Despite these caveats, I still recommend and support the eating of reasonably good quality animal protein. Where possible, grass-fed beef, free-range or organic poultry, as well as non-farmed fish. Just keep in mind that you need to watch the quantities.

Protein requirements

While excess protein is bad for you, it is important to consume an adequate amount of protein on a daily basis. The question is: how much is enough?

Various authorities have produced guidelines, which are normally based around a 'healthy' quantity of grams of protein per kilogram of body mass. In the U.S., the official RDA (Recommended Daily Allowance) has been set to 0.8 grams of protein per kilogram of body mass for the average person. You can approximate this value to 1 gram per kilogram to make calculation easier, but remember that it does overstate requirements. If you carry extra body fat, this will also tend to overstate your actual requirements.

In general most people, even the fairly active, will require between 50 and 100 grams of protein daily – at most.

Watch your protein intake!

Use these guidelines as an easy way to estimate the amount of protein in the food you eat:

- Meat and chicken are about 50% protein
- Cheese is about 50% protein
- Fish varies between 35% and 60% protein (tuna)
- Eggs are about 25% protein
- Milk is less than 10% and cream is less than 5%

Eat sensibly. Don't eat animal protein more than once a day and when you do, try to limit your portion size to 150 grams or less. Also try to eat more fatty portions when you can and try not to eat animal protein every day.

Animal vs. plant protein

The evolved Banting diet proposed in this book caters easily for vegetarians and vegans because it has a more relaxed attitude to carb intake. This is not the case when Banting, which is difficult for vegetarians and all but impossible for vegans because of the relatively high carb content of many vegetarian/vegan foods. It is also a struggle to find foods that are high enough in fat, especially under a vegan diet.

When it comes to protein, it is more difficult for vegetarians and vegans to source complete protein, and it also requires a greater volume of food to be consumed to reach daily protein requirements. This leaves vegetarians and vegans with a greatly reduced risk of protein overconsumption.

Complete protein sources for vegetarians and vegans are available despite being less convenient than animal protein. These include chlorella, hemp seeds, chia seeds, and quinoa. Soy is also an option; it has a high protein content but is much more open to contamination with pesticides and about 90% of all soy is GMO modified. There are also concerns that it contains estrogen-based hormone disruptors.

CHAPTER 9

REDUCING INSULIN — THE HARD WAY

'Doc if you want to find a butter knife and
start carving on me now, let's do it!'
bariatricgirl.com

Towards the end of 2011, a story was published about a trio of petite sisters who were taken to lunch by a journalist in a quiet Pennsylvania restaurant. As you no doubt know, a journalist only pays for lunch when there's a big story to be told. Big it was, but not at the time they ordered lunch; by then, each of the sisters had managed to lose half of herself.

In the recent past, they had collectively weighed over 350 kilograms, enough heft to play see-saw with the three hulks manning the front row of a national rugby team. Between them, they had tried every kind of diet, weight loss pill or get-lean supplement on the planet. All of which had done naught to slow their relentless weight gain.

Amazingly, in 2002, the youngest sister found a cure; a miracle that worked for them all. It evaporated their excess fat and landed them a lunch with the journalist, with the three of them looking like a gaggle of mature models for a chic range of New York clothing.

It was not a diet that delivered them from the sea of fat they were drowning in; it was something much more drastic. They had their stomachs stapled by a bariatric surgeon and their lives changed for better and for worse as a consequence.

Bariatric surgery

As we have learned from the three skinny sisters, provided that you survive the operation with no complications, surgery is a fail-safe way to lose weight and lower insulin levels. Bariatric surgery is the fancy name for operations designed to produce weight loss. Better known as stomach stapling, these operations will visibly transform most patients within six months to a year. Other important chemical changes occur more quickly. In as little as four weeks post-op, previously deranged blood chemistry returns to normal as insulin sensitivity is restored and diabetes is reversed.

This, dear reader, is your pot of gold at the end of the rainbow; your real goal. It's easy to get distracted by the big weight loss but the real benefit comes from the effect that these operations have on diabetes and insulin levels.

If you're ever in the market for a gastric bypass operation, which I sincerely hope never happens, you will find that there are a number of surgical options. It's a little like choosing a new car where you have to balance cost against convenience and resale value.

Roo-On-Why

The sisters went for the most popular, famous version of bariatric surgery, called the Roux-En-Y procedure. Its name is pronounced like the title above. The Roux-En-Y and its variations permanently reduce the size of the stomach. As you can see in the diagram overleaf, most of the stomach has been bypassed. The remaining portion of the stomach and a short loop of small intestine are left in place.

The operation places a hard physical limit to the quantity of food that can be consumed at one sitting. As soon as too much food is eaten, it stops going down and bubbles over like a bath with a blocked drain.

Roux-en-Y
esophago-jejunostomy

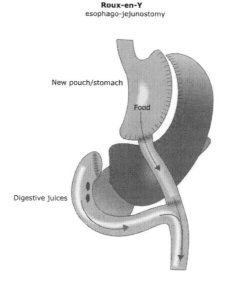

New pouch/stomach

Food

Digestive juices

If a permanent change sounds too drastic, there are other non-permanent methods available to reduce stomach size. In gastric banding for example, the surgeon places an adjustable band around the stomach through a small keyhole incision. This has the advantage of allowing the stomach size to be adjusted from the outside via a small port on the skin.

However, before you start fantasising about having this kind of operation, there are a few gotchas that may put you off a little.

Bariatric gotchas

The effects of waking up from surgery with a stomach that had a part as an extra in the movie 'Honey I Shrunk the kids', are profound. The owner of this new downsized organ will quickly find out that it fills quicker than a teacup and is no longer the black hole that was there previously. Reduced capacity is just one little problem. Other issues soon appear such as gagging on the smell or the taste of foods that previously delighted.

Eating a seemingly innocuous morsel can also cause unexpected problems. For example, one of the three sisters, who in the past had hoovered down chocolate malt balls by the bagful, now had a two-malt-ball limit. Then not long after they went down, these two critters 'repeated' on her, causing vicious heart palpitations. This well-known complication of stapling is called 'dumping', which is caused when foods that cannot be properly digested in the stomach are 'dumped' into the small intestine, causing abdominal distress.

Not so fast...

While bariatric operations produce startling weight loss in almost 100% of cases, the effects do not always last. Most of the weight reduction happens in the first year, which is usually maintained until the end of the second year. By five years post-op, more than 80% of patients will have regained about half of the weight they had lost and an astounding 10% will return to their initial weight!

The main reason behind this weight gain seems to be the slow and steady enlargement of the stomach, which is probably caused by persistent over-eating behaviour.

Lessons from bariatric surgery

For most of us, bariatric surgery is not an option. Firstly because it is reserved for the truly obese and then, more tellingly, because of its multiple negative outcomes: the risks of having the operation, the extended post-op recovery period as well as the life-altering eating discomfort.

However, we can learn something really important from the results of this kind of surgery; these operations abruptly restrict food intake which leads to an almost immediate lowering of insulin levels and the steady normalisation of insulin sensitivity.

Wouldn't it be amazing if there was a way for us to reap the benefits of bariatric surgery, without having the operation? There is – and I will tell you about it in the next chapter.

CHAPTER 10

REDUCING INSULIN — THE EASY WAY

'Hunger is a necessary nutrient.'
Nassim Taleb – Ancestral Health Symposium (2013)

It may be hard to believe but not that long ago, a team of doctors surpassed the food reduction of stomach stapling and created an environment that starved a young patient to death. This tragedy played out against the backdrop of a belief in Victorian England that the ability to survive without eating was a sign of spiritual purity. During this time, four pre-adolescent girls, who came to be known as The Victorian Fasting Girls, rose to fame and were revered as the 'supermodels' of their day.

One them was Sarah Jacobs. She began to abstain from eating at age nine, when she found that fasting cured the uncontrollable convulsions she suffered from. News of the miracle began to spread when her parents let it be known that their daughter remained in peak health despite not eating. People began to journey to the small village where they lived in rural Wales to witness this miracle for themselves. They brought money and gifts which they laid around Sarah's bed.

Over time, bathed as she was in such attention, Sarah began to look a little too well for the liking of some visitors who reported that she had 'plump and pinky cheeks'. This led to speculation about the veracity of the miracle and a committee of doctors from Guy's Hospital in London became involved in a genuine effort to prove that the miracle was real. Amid much excitement, a team of trained nurses was sent to institute an around-the-clock watch to ensure that Sarah neither ate nor drank anything. As a safety precaution, Sarah was instructed to ask for food if she wanted, but she did not.

For seven days, Sarah weakened as doctors made notes and her parents stood by wringing their hands. Finally, following a series of convulsions, she lapsed into a coma and died. Later, when they autopsied her body, the bones of a small sparrow where found in her stomach. The public were outraged and fingered her parents for her death. They were both tried and sent to prison for manslaughter. Shamefully, the doctors and nurses who had attended to Sarah's death were absolved of all blame.

While Sarah's tragic outcome is something we need to avoid, one thing we can be sure of is that her insulin sensitivity was really high. Acts of lunacy aside, surely there is some middle ground between the surgical stapling of stomachs and the total abstinence of The Victorian Fasting Girls.

Let's get to IF

There is a much simpler and ultimately more effective alternative to having surgery to reduce insulin resistance. It's called fasting.

Today, fasting as an occasional tool for weight loss has become known as Intermittent Fasting. Used correctly, Intermittent Fasting (IF) is a powerful tool against excessive insulin levels. With IF, you can avoid the invasive surgery of stomach stapling, the months of gastric rehabilitation and a lifetime of eating discomfort. IF can deliver better and more lasting results without the surgery; at the same time it can transform overall health and extend lifespan.

Many people panic when I bring up the subject of fasting. 'Doc, how can I possibly go without eating, I spend all day dreaming about my next meal?'

Fasting is easier than it sounds. When combined with a reduction in sugar intake, using my version of relaxed Banting, the sensation of hunger becomes greatly reduced or even vanishes completely.

Outcomes of fasting

Before you toss this book in the bin or switch off your E-reader, allow me a few minutes to convince you that fasting can change your life.

Do any of these outcomes interest you?
- Want more energy? FAST
- Want to think more clearly? FAST
- Want to look younger? FAST
- Want to lose weight? FAST
- Want to age slower? FAST
- Want to live longer? FAST
- Want to have better sex? FAST

If that list does not get you going, then I give up. Throw the book away or switch off your E-reader. Otherwise, listen up!

What I aim to teach you is a relaxed form of Banting that is combined with a precision form of Intermittent Fasting. Together they form a power tool that will reduce insulin levels and increase insulin sensitivity. Employed correctly, my method will produce lasting weight loss in almost anyone, including women over forty and those becalmed by weight loss plateaus.

Fast? Me? Are you crazy?

If you are anything like my average patient, the mere thought of skipping breakfast is a daunting prospect. Maybe not eating for an entire day seems a little crazy. Initially, I thought the idea was crazy too, but bear with me because our bodies are designed to work brilliantly without food and you will be surprised how easy it can really be.

For a better grasp of just how well our bodies are designed to run on water alone for extended periods, let's look at our in-built human experience, a legacy that has evolved over the last 100,000 years.

Ancestral thinking

Our ancestors certainly did not have a regular food supply. They had no supermarkets or bar fridges and they started every day on an empty stomach.

The sun would wake them to their primary task; find food for the day! On most days, food would not be conveniently lying around waiting for them to eat it. Each meal required work: a walk to find it; a struggle to catch it; a battle to carry it; and time to prepare it. Often their search for food would compel them to enter hostile territory on empty stomachs.

Dangerous terrain and hunger are the key here, because humans don't stand a chance against any half-serious predator. In order to survive we had to evolve to be on top of our game when we were hungry. Today we don't access these skills; instead when we get hungry we get irritable, short-tempered and make silly mistakes. In ancestral times, you would soon turn into a take-away dinner if you tramped around the bush hungry, irritable and partially alert.

When we eat we become lazy and content, which is precisely why we are designed to be at our strongest mentally and physically when we are hungry and running on stored body fat; otherwise we would not be here as a species today.

Try it! It's an in-built skill that is waiting to be put to work for you in the same way it worked for our ancestors. When you are fasting, you will be at your best and anyone who messes with you had better watch out! Abstaining from eating puts you into a state of maximum 'aliveness', which is probably why so many religions, old and new, revere the fasting state.

Religious fasting

Fasting is an important aspect of many religions. Some Native American tribes used fasting during vision quests where they tried to communicate with guardian spirits. Ancient Greeks used fasting as a means of healing themselves and today, fasting is an important part of many modern religions. Buddhism, Hinduism, Christianity, Judaism and Islam all have periods of food abstinence associated with rituals and rules.

Most of these rituals seek some form of transcendence from the physical restraints of the human body, which is facilitated by fasting. A sense of wellbeing often seems to accompany periods of fasting. (There are sound medical reasons for this – more about these later.) Some religions revere longer fasts, especially for their holy leaders who are sometimes said to have survived extended periods of abstinence from food and even water.

The question is, how long is a long fast?

The longest fast

If you had to fast for an extended period, drinking only unsweetened fluids like water, black tea or black coffee, how long do you think you could last? A day or two? Could you ever contemplate something as seemingly impossible as a traditional 40-day water fast?

Do you think it's possible to fast for a year?

How about 382 days? That's how long Mr A.B., an obese 27-year-old patient at the University Department of Medicine in Dundee, Scotland, in 1973, managed to maintain a supervised fast. He drank only water and unsweetened tea and took no supplements besides a daily multivitamin pill. His fast transformed him from a 207-kilogram heavyweight to a svelte 82 kilos at the end. He functioned normally throughout and regular tests showed that his blood chemistry remained completely normal. Initially he had no intention of fasting for over a year, but he felt so well that his medical advisors allowed him to continue. At the end of his fast, they reported that 'Prolonged fasting in this patient had no ill effect'.

Once again, don't panic, I am not proposing that you fast for any period longer than a day!

Before we get to the How To details, let's take a look at some of the benefits and debunk some of the myths of fasting.

CHAPTER 11

FASTING: BENEFITS AND MYTHS

'Humans live on one-quarter of what they eat;
on the other three-quarters live their doctor.'
6,000-year-old Egyptian pyramid inscription (3,800 BC)

The benefits of fasting

Fasting is a powerful tool that will give health benefits you will actually be able to feel. On fasting days, you will brim with extra energy and your mind will be noticeably sharper. Fast regularly for a few weeks and you will feel the difference; you will shed excess weight and will look younger.

As much as these claims sound like marketing hype, they are not. They are backed up by a stack of research papers as well as a legion of personal experiences. Fasting improves mind and body in many ways. Over the last few years, there has been a flood of good news about the benefits of fasting. By way of example, a recent study by Professor Valter Longo, Professor of Gerontology at the University of Southern California, showed that a fasting diet slowed aging in a group of subjects within a period as short as a few months.

Here are some of the benefits you can expect from your new intermittent fasting lifestyle:

- Kills hunger
- Reduces insulin levels

- Increases fat burning
- Increases energy and 'feel good' mood
- Increases growth hormone
- Slows aging
- Boosts brain power
- Prevents Alzheimer's

Kills hunger

While you may be hungry when you first try it, once you get used to doing it you will find that fasting kills your hunger. It seems to work for everyone; hunger disappears after a few days or weeks of pangs. Many people report that eating seems to make them more hungry over the course of a day while not eating seems to do the opposite. I personally find that when I start a day with breakfast, I think about eating all day and will happily eat just about anything that is put in front of me. This does not happen at all on my fasting days.

Reduced insulin levels and increased insulin sensitivity

Insulin levels begin to drop a few hours after a meal and they remain low until food is next eaten. The longer the time between meals, the more sensitive cells become to insulin. This is the core drive of intermittent fasting; mixing occasional fasting days with normal eating days that, over time, leads to restored insulin sensitivity.

As you will see in the next chapter, there are many ways to separate normal eating days with fasting days. The exact scheduling is up to you and you can adjust it to suit your personal preference and convenience.

Increased fat burning

Stroll through the aisles of slimming products or the nutrition section of your local pharmacy and you will quickly lose count of the number of products claiming to speed up fat-burning and metabolism. These kinds of products are usually emblazoned with marketing slogans that promise to get rid of body fat; 'fat burner', 'thermo lean', 'belly blaster', and 'lipo shredder'. Sadly, the better these potions work, the more potential they have to cause health issues like anxiety, high blood pressure, gastric upsets, heart palpitations and more.

Whether they work or not, all fat-burning potions and lotions cost money. Hang onto your wallet! Fasting saves money and always burns fat; no side-effects, risks or guesswork required. It is beyond doubt that fasting leads to fat burning; this has been medically verified and proved in multiple studies over the last hundred years. Critically, fasting preserves muscle and bone mass, while low-calorie dieting has been shown to produce the opposite effect.

Fasting also saves you the time of procuring or preparing the food for the meals you skip; think of the time and cost saved if you gave up eating breakfast and lunch a few times a week. Which option sounds better to you? A no-cost certainty or some dubious potion that produces expensive urine?

Increased energy and 'feel good' mood

Fasting causes a beneficial, gradual rise in adrenaline levels. This slow rise of adrenaline is not at all like the sharp, sudden spike of adrenaline that hits you when you are startled or afraid. Fasting's job is to facilitate glucose release from fat stores, otherwise called fat-burning! However, higher levels of adrenaline have other more palpable effects: an increase in energy levels, a happier mood, better memory and sharpened attention. Don't be surprised if fasting makes you feel upbeat and energized.

Increased growth hormone levels

Fasting naturally increases growth hormone (GH) levels, which is really good news because GH is intimately involved with regeneration and cell growth.

Our GH levels drop as we pass out of our twenties and keep getting lower as we grow older. Giving middle-aged people more GH makes them look and feel younger and physically stronger. When used on the sports field, GH turbocharges athletes, making them faster and stronger. In the gym, GH is the go-to drug for bodybuilders looking to build bigger muscles.

These are some of the reasons why people try to get their hands on GH through their doctors or by accessing semi-legal or illegal channels. The result of this demand has led to adult GH sales that vastly outweigh prescriptions for children of short stature, which is its originally intended market. In 2004 for example, 74% of all GH prescribed in America went to adult patients. This is a shocking example of the greed of Big Pharma turning a blind eye as profits roll in, not least because a known side-effect of adults injecting GH is an increased cancer risk.

Despite these risks, the motivation to be bigger, stronger or faster seems to override common sense. I recently consulted a 55-year-old cyclist, a vegan for religious reasons, who was looking for nutritional advice to help him ride faster than his cycling buddies. During our consultation he let slip that he was spending enoughbuying GH injections to feed a family of four each month.

There is no need to spend exorbitant amounts or to go to illegal or desperate lengths to raise your GH levels. Fasting can do it for you, safely and legally.

Slower aging

Fasting decreases inflammation and oxidative stress throughout the body and thus slows the rate the body ages.

Without getting too technical, oxidative stress is like rust on a car. As our bodies age, so we accumulate oxidation damage (rust), caused by the free radicals that are produced by our cells. While this cannot be avoided and is a natural consequence of living, some activities and eating patterns unnecessarily increase oxidation damage. Many anti-aging formulas and vita-min products are designed to reduce this kind of damage but choosing a product off the shelves of your local health store is a hit-or-miss affair. Why bother when fasting has been proved to work?

Fasting not only reduces free radical production, it also slows the rate of cell deterioration by increasing the expression of the genetic pathways that delay aging. These claims are not just marketing phrases! They have been repeatedly verified by experiment. For example, it is well known that we can increase the lifespan of certain lab animals by over 30% simply by reducing their food intake. These findings are applicable to humans too; increased longevity trends are common in religious sects that fast for long periods or restrict food intake.

These benefits are more than likely a result of reduced free radical generation caused by lower food intake, coupled with lower average insulin levels.

Fasting and your brain

Fasting does amazing things to our brains. These effects can be divided into two; immediate brain power boosting effects and long-term protective effects. Both of which we have great use for.

Boosting brain power

The fasting state seems to produce clarity of thought that is completely different to the woozy post-meal thought process we are all so familiar with. Chemically, it is clear why this happens; under fasting conditions, the brain switches over from using sugars as its primary energy source to run on ketones, which are fat-based. Some scientists believe, as do I, that ketones are the preferred energy source for the brain and that our modern diet forces our brains to switch to burning glucose. This makes running a brain on glucose equivalent to running a petrol-engine car on diesel fuel.

Fasting will improve your memory!

It works for lab animals and it will work for you. Tests show that fasting mice perform significantly better than normal when tasked with tests of memory and learning like maze-running. Like this report: 'Mice on intermittent fasting had better learning and memory assessed by the Barnes maze and fear conditioning'. (Liaoliao Li, Zhi Wang, Zhiyi Zuo Department of Anaesthesiology, University of Virginia, Charlottesville, May 2013.)

Anti-degenerative effects

As we age, our brains are in great danger. The longer we live, the harder it becomes to avoid degenerative diseases of the brain like the universally feared Alzheimer's disease. Cases of Alzheimer's disease are mushrooming and are predicted to triple in the next 30 years. Even today, almost every second senior in America who reaches 80 years old will develop Alzheimer's. Distressingly, this disease affects two-thirds more women than men.

The good news is that lab studies have shown that fasting either prevents or slows the progress of many brain degenerative diseases. Professor Mark Mattson, who works at the John Hopkins School of Medicine in Baltimore, Maryland, USA, has modelled diseases like Alzheimer's and Parkinson's in his lab and has found that energy restriction in the form of intermittent fasting slows and even prevents these diseases in his experimental mice. Mattson firmly believes that intermittent fasting will have a similar effect in humans.

Busting some fasting myths

Stoking the fire: One of the most persistent nutrition myths maintains that we need to eat regularly to stoke the fire of our metabolism. Fasting puts the body into 'emergency mode' which then causes a reduction in energy output, similar to the behaviour of an electronic device going into low-power hibernation mode.

This is nonsense. If our ancestors' systems worked like this, we would have died out as a species thousands of years ago. In reality, the opposite happens and fasting increases metabolic rate; this occurs in fasts that last a day or longer, as well as alternate day fasting.

Low blood sugar: People often claim that they become shaky and weak from a lack of food, which they blame on low blood sugar levels.

Really? Just how likely is it that a normal body would keel over from lack of sugar? If this was a real problem, the sight of people collapsing on sidewalks and drivers going off the road from blood sugar lows would be commonplace. Our bodies are exquisitely engineered to maintain stable blood sugar levels, irrespective of whether we have eaten or not.

A good example is our 328-day faster, Mr A.B., who was never troubled by low blood sugar during his fast. He reported that he felt energised and his blood sugar levels, which were regularly tested, remained normal for the entire year that he fasted. Fasting will work for you as well and low blood sugar is highly unlikely to trouble you when you fast. While it is possible that you may experience some discomfort when you stop eating, this will soon pass, as the 100,000 years of experience engineered into your body kicks in to ensure that your blood sugar levels remain stable.

Hunger control: The 'six small meals a day' dogma is another myth that seems to have a life of its own. This eating strategy represents the polar opposite of fasting or a single-meal day, which is something I strongly advocate. Eating six times a day ensures that insulin levels remain raised all day, a completely undesirable effect. In addition, hunger is not suppressed. Fasting, on the other hand, quickly suppresses hunger, lowers insulin levels and clears the head, allowing for much more productive days, uninterrupted by time off preparing and eating multiple meals.

Muscle loss: Another mistaken belief is that irregular eating results in a loss of muscle and bone mass; this contradicts medical research. Despite the fact that a number of studies have shown that low-calorie diets lead to the loss of muscle and bone, the same cannot be said for fasting. This means that the 'eat a little less' approach, recommended by so many health professionals, is not the way to go.

You eat more when you fast: This is actually true. Studies show that people do actually eat a bit more when breaking a fast. However, it is not possible to eat enough to make up for the lost time.

A study done on alternate-day fasting showed that despite somewhat higher calorie intake on non-fasting days, this strategy produced an energy deficit of about 2,000 calories over every two-day cycle. This calorie deficit adds up and, over time, will produce significant weight loss. Contrast this to a diet that restricts calories, which reduces energy intake by a similar amount, but causes the body to switch to a lower metabolic state.

I hope that by now I have convinced you to consider the fasting option.

Fasting is not nearly as hard as it looks … all you have to do is trust yourself.

CHAPTER 12
FOUNDATIONS OF FASTING

'As soon as you trust yourself, you will know how to live.'
Goethe

Once upon a time, a young man was walking in Paris when he heard a familiar tune. He stopped in his tracks, unable to believe his ears. Coming from behind the door of the club he had just walked past was his tune. Literally his tune, not just a piece of music he was emotionally attached to. He had composed it and now, incredibly, it was being performed in Paris.

Seven years before, our young man had approached a small Montevideo orchestra to play the tango he wrote. He had just completed it and couldn't wait to hear it played but had been too shy to put his name to it. Unknown to him, the tune had become popular in Uruguay and had migrated to Paris, from where it would spread around the world. Today, *La Comparsita* is the most famous tango tune in the world. Gerardo Rodriguez, its young composer, spent most of his adult life trying to regain ownership of it.

Before we learn a little more about how to approach fasting, realise this: fasting itself is not hard. The hard part is conquering the fear of not eating. Getting up in the morning and leaving home on an empty stomach is a scary prospect for many people.

It certainly was for me, but it can be overcome as long as you trust yourself and your body.

The story about *La Comparsita* is a classic case of a talented person without sufficient trust in himself. Think how much more productive as a composer Rodriguez could have been if he had not wasted so much time and energy on legal battles?

Trust yourself to leave home without eating and, after the difficulties of the first few times, and as many others have discovered, you will find it liberating. You will soon discover the value of not having to serve the whims of your hunger and you will enjoy having more time and energy to devote to your day.

Many people behave as if their bodies have a physical need to be topped-up with food all day in order to function properly. This is nonsense. A lot of the time, people eat because of boredom, habit or as part of a routine. They respond to social pressures to eat at certain times even though hunger is absent and there is no physical requirement to eat.

Breaking the breakfast habit

Skipping breakfast is the gateway to easy fasting. As I mentioned in an earlier chapter on insulin resistance, the phrase 'breakfast is the most important meal of the day', which originated from the Kellogg's cornflake empire, has become a truth unto itself. It has become embedded in our social fabric and is spouted by medical professionals and marketing folk as if it's a moral certainty.

Unfortunately, reality and fiction don't always reconcile. Our ancestors didn't wake up to a bowl of muesli and yogurt served on the patio. Instead, they faced the day on an empty stomach with a need to fill it before sunset. Because of this ancient cycle, we have inherited the ability to run on empty for extended periods of time. It just takes time for our bodies to 'remember' how to run on reserve fuel and, at the same time, to eradicate the breakfast habit.

Here is an example that may help you to visualise how you could go about making breakfast optional. Meet Salamina, a beautiful middle-aged woman, who cleans the office in a business I visit from time to time. Over a few years of trading pleasantries, we have come to learn a little about each other's lives. Salamina knows I have three kids whom I dote on and she occasionally shares some news about her two boys. She works a long day, bookended by a two-hour journey to and from work. She lives alone and wakes at 4 am to prepare breakfast and lunch for her day. The long walk to her bus gives her no time to eat at home, so she breakfasts at work before the office staff arrive. During the day, she also drinks a few cups of sugary tea.

One day she confided in me that she had been told by a doctor at her clinic that she was overweight and needed to lose 30 kilograms; they also wanted her to start on treatment for diabetes.

'Will you let me help you?' I asked. She nodded, so I went on, 'There are only two things I need you to do.'

'No more breakfast and no more sugar.'

She gladly agreed to drop the sugar in her tea but was adamant that she did too much physical work to cope without breakfast. I suggested a simple strategy; that she eat breakfast an hour later each week until she could combine it with her lunch. To this she agreed and two months passed before we met again in her office reception. Her smile greeted me before I could say hello. Pulling me into the small kitchen that served as her office, she told me her weight was down enough to make her clothes loose and that she was only eating lunch every day.

'What about supper?' I asked.

'I don't have time to make it, I just get home, bath and go straight to bed.'

She said her lunch was now her only daily meal and she was feeling so much better that she was beginning to enjoy the long walk to her bus in the mornings.

What we can learn from Salamina is that all it takes is a little gumption and some self-belief to change a way of life. Think creatively about how you could remove breakfast from your routine; there is always a way if you are committed. However you look at it, learning to fast, starting with skipping breakfast and then working up to skipping lunch as well, is much easier than getting a surgeon to staple your stomach. And as you have read in the previous chapter, fasting will give you better results than surgery. If you learn to trust yourself, you can achieve amazing things.

Of course, if you feel that you can handle big changes, then do it cold turkey! Either way, cold turkey or slow and sure, get rid of breakfast and you will be on the road to better health and more energy.

Fasting windows

There are many formulas for fasting which you can adjust to suit your needs. You can also change and adapt new fasting routines as your lifestyle changes. There are two types of fasts: 'fasting windows' and long-term fasts. Fasting windows are shorter periods, measured in hours; long-term fasts usually last days, weeks or months.

Initially, I suggest that you start with a short, flexible fasting window that suits your lifestyle. As you learn how to adapt to not eating, you can 'open' or 'close' your fasting window as you need to. Eventually you will settle on a schedule that works for you.

The shortest practical fasting window is the period that starts when you go to sleep at night until you wake in the morning. This gives you an approximate 12-hour fast which is broken when you eat breakfast. Some people naturally don't feel hungry when they wake up and find skipping breakfast easy to do. If you are like this great, otherwise try to push out the time that you eat your breakfast by a few hours. Then once you get used to your new breakfast time, keep eating it later and later in the morning, until you can make it to lunchtime which will give you a 16 to 18-hour window. Then, gradually push your lunch time later and later in the afternoon, until you can make it all the way to dinnertime without eating.

Fasting for the whole day gives you a 24-hour fasting window, which is the most practical period for short fasts. Breaking your fast at dinnertime allows you to eat with family or friends and has good social benefits. This is my preferred method; it leaves me with extra time and energy during the day because I don't have to waste time on finding and eating food. Also after a short while (usually three to six weeks), you will no longer feel hungry during your fasting window and you will soon start appreciating how much the lack of this need simplifies your life.

Another approach is the 36-hour fast where you go to bed without eating, fast the whole of the following day and only eat again the following morning.

It is important not to become too rigid and allow yourself to break a fast occasionally, for example if you feel unusually hungry or if a social occasion demands it. There is always another day and we all need to break rules from time to time!

Some commercial examples

A number of popular lifestyles or diets use a fasting window as their 'shtick' or marketing gimmick. Interestingly, quite a few of these diets have an athletic, training or bodybuilding basis. One of the earliest is the Warrior Diet by Ori Hofmeckler. It is based on a hypothetical Stone Age warrior or worker who is assumed to have consumed little, if any, food during a day that comprised a fair amount of physical activity. The warrior then ate his single daily meal at night in a so-called 'over-feeding' phase, resulting in a fasting window of approximately 20 hours. The Warrior Diet also stresses the eating of non-processed, organic foods and allows both high-fat and high-carb meals, with the strange proviso that carbs be eaten last during a meal so as to help stabilise insulin levels.

Another example with bodybuilding roots is Eat Stop Eat by Brad Pilon. It too embodies a day of intermittent fasting once or twice a week. The diet's founder has obviously benefitted from the diet and proudly displays pictures of himself in bodybuilding poses. The diet misses some of the benefits of intermittent fasting for insulin reduction because it prohibits more than a single fasting day at a time. The most likely reason for this is to preserve muscle mass, but current research would contradict this and I think that multiple fasting days are perfectly fine in the right circumstances.

More recently, The 5:2 Diet has become prominent after being popularized by Dr Michael Mosley, a well-known BBC television journalist. His best-selling book, *The Fast Diet*, written with journalist Mimi Spencer (Atria Books) proposed a routine of five days of normal eating mixed with two days of reduced calorie intake, called fasting days. Mosley suggests that men should restrict themselves to 600 calories on fasting days, while women make do with 500 calories. These restrictions are effectively a quarter of the generally accepted average daily calories for men and women respectively. Theoretically, dieters on the 5:2 should decrease their total weekly calorie consumption by about 3,000 calories a week which means that if they don't grossly overeat on normal eating days, they will lose weight over time.

My issue with the 5:2 Diet is the way meals are structured on fasting days. The diet protocol accommodates (and suggests) the splitting of meals on fasting days, allowing for a small breakfast and a small lunch or supper. Used this way, the diet can still produce weight loss because of the calorie deficit but it will not address the more important issue of increasing insulin sensitivity. This can only be properly achieved with longer periods of zero calorie intake, allowing basal insulin levels to drop for a reasonable period of 16 to 20 hours on some days of the week.

The 'diet' I suggest in this book is similar but not the same as these examples. (See next chapter for details.)

Longer fasts

Beyond the 36-hour fasting window are the fasts that extend for days. As we read earlier, there is really no physical limit to how long you can fast as long as you carry the necessary body fat to sustain it and you drink sufficient fluids. The more fat you carry, the longer you can sustain a fast and the better your results will be.

Time and patience

Remember that it takes time to chew up any body fat that you may carry. You can only reasonably sustain long fasts if you carry the weight in the first place. Muscle and bone follow when most of your fat has been burned, which is not at all desirable for your general health.

Fasting and training

Fasting and training work well together. Some people find that they become weak or shaky when they first begin exercising on an empty stomach but this feeling normally passes. If it happens to you, try to have a small bite or a drink to get you over the unpleasant feeling but try to persevere when next you train.

I suggest that you regard training as a normal part of your day and unless you are bodybuilding or engaged in long periods of endurance training, you should simply train on water; you should have no need for any sports drinks, energy bars or protein shakes.

(You can read why training while fasting increases weight loss in the chapter You Lie! Eat Less, Exercise More, towards the end of this book.)

Fasting fluids

When you fast, you must drink as often and as freely as you need to.

You can drink as much as you want of any unsweetened liquids, hot or cold. This includes water, sparking or still, as well as black tea or coffee. It may make it easier for you to add a small amount of cream or milk to your coffee to take the bite off it. You can also add a little milk to your tea but be careful with quantities. I recently met a patient for coffee while he was on a fasting day and was surprised to see him empty the contents of his cream container into his black coffee. If you need a measure, use no more than a tablespoon of cream or full-cream milk.

Sugar is obviously not allowed and I strongly suggest that no artificial sweeteners are used. Many people use sweeteners as an alternative to sugar but they are addictive and are difficult to stop cold turkey. If you find that you cannot tolerate an imme-diate end to your diet drink intake, use a strategy of progressively diluting your drink with water to wean yourself off it.

Clear bone broth soups are another alternative. You can make these with any soup broth base like vegetables, chicken or meat and then drink them hot or cold.

Those who should not fast

Fasting is a brilliant health tool but it is not for everyone! Some people should not fast; pregnant or breastfeeding mothers, children, or anyone who is too thin already. People with eating disorders need to be especially cautious because fasting may worsen existing eating patterns. In general, people suffering from chronic debilitating diseases as well as those who are malnourished should not fast.

While most type 2 diabetics can benefit from careful adoption of fasting, type 1 diabetics are a special case. It is possible for them to fast but it requires special precautions; I have outlined a possible strategy for type 1s in the Appendix of this book – Fasting for type 1 diabetics.

That said, fasting is good medicine for most of us.

Let's outline some fasting strategies you can adopt to suit yourself and banish Banting forever.

CHAPTER 13

BANTING BEGONE!

'Are you not dead? Begone!'

I think it is time to throw out the concept of Banting in its current popular format. Let us replace it with a better way to Bant that combines intermittent fasting with relaxed carb rules, while retaining the principles of no calorie counting or food weighing.

Banting has outlived its 100-year history. In its modern guise, it bans an entire food group and is applied in ways that become too obsessive and restrictive. Banting results in a diet that is heavily weighted in favour of fat and protein. Excess fat consumption is probably not bad for us but excess protein certainly is.

Because of its obsessive carb avoidance, Banting's long-term appeal is limited to a handful of devotees who almost cherish its restrictions and can maintain the faith for an extended period; these are usually the same kind of people who earn max points for gym attendance! For the rest of us, the boredom of high-fat meals soon sets in, prompting small transgressions which, over time, result in the dreaded carb creep. This almost inevitable falling off the wagon then leads to the slow but inevitable regain of weight lost.

Doing things differently

In order to succeed, we have to do things differently!

We need to better utilise our highly adaptable digestive system that has evolved to enable us to thrive on a wide variety of different foods sourced from any geographical location on the planet. What we need is a reasonable diet that lies between the extremes of the fat-eating Eskimos and the island-locked Okinawans living on a diet of almost pure carbs.

Surely, somewhere between the extremes of the 'low-carb, high-fat diets' and 'high-carb, low-fat diets', we can find a solution that works more comfortably for us?

I believe the more reasonable solution is one that removes neither carbs nor fat as entire food groups and accepts that pure high-fat diets or extremely low-carb diets are not good for anyone in the long term.

Balancing energy

To our new approach, which allows a relaxed attitude to carbs and consequently a more balanced approach to our food choices, let's add the following:

The intake of excessive energy, particularly when caused by incessant eating and snacking, is the root cause of our health and overweight issues.

It is the consequence of incessant eating and the resulting excess energy intake that causes insulin resistance, which is then followed by a cascade of health issues.

When we start to control our energy intake, using intermittent fasting, we CAN add carbs to our diet.

To summarise:

- Overeating causes overweight.

- Once gained, excess weight is difficult to lose.

- Excess weight can be lost using the Banting diet, which severely restricts carbs.

- Alternatively, excess weight can be lost more effectively using intermittent fasting, which balances periods of reduced energy intake with periods of normal energy intake in a more natural way and works with established evolutionary mechanisms.

- Intermittent fasting allows us to eat a more relaxed diet on non-fasting days.

Therefore, provided that we try our best to eat real food and to avoid processed foods and sugar, we can eat pretty much anything we like on non-fasting days.

Does that sound like a good deal? A trade-off between some days where you eat very little and others where you can eat freely?

Let's look at a new deal in dieting...

CHAPTER 14

A NEW DEAL

'By rights you're a king. If I was you, I'd call for a new deal.'
O. Henry

Let's put it all together and call for a new deal on diet. Something simpler, less restrictive, healthier, and easier to live with than Banting or LCHF.

Here's the deal:

- **Carbs,** especially in their natural form, are allowed; this includes some bread, fruit, rice, oats, potatoes, and some other previously banned carbs.

- **Protein,** animal or vegetable, is allowed but should be limited in quantity or frequency to reduce its aging and cancer-promoting effects.

- **Fats** are encouraged as long as they come from a natural source.

- **Fasting** on some days comprising of, at most, a single meal in a 24-hour cycle.

- Processed foods must be avoided when possible.

If you do nothing else…

- **Fast for 20 to 24 hours twice a week, drinking only unsweetened fluids.**

- **Eat three meals per day for the rest of the week, but eat moderately and follow the guidelines contained in this book.**

That's all it takes and the deal will work for you.

You could theoretically continue to eat junk food, add sugar to your drinks and keep snacking between meals on non-fasting days and it should still work for weight loss. However, it would be foolhardy to do this as it will take longer for the weight to come off and you will miss out on the real benefits to your health. The method I recommend still fixes one important aspect of diets like the 5:2 Diet; it ensures an extended fasting window and allows insulin levels to drop meaningfully.

Done this way, the diet will perform like a sports car that is used to take chickens to market; it will still work but much of its true performance potential will remain untapped.

The IF (intermittent fasting) eating plan will work better for you if your fasts are combined with non-fasting days where you eat non-processed natural food, avoid sugar and don't snack between meals. This way, you will witness major improvements to your health over the long term. Eating healthy, non-processed foods is the hardest part because it requires restraint: saying NO to junk food and being selective about the food you put into your body is hard work.

Foods to be avoided

Let's start with a list of forbidden stuff and get the hard part out of the way. While these items should not be part of any healthy diet, life still needs to be lived! An occasional slip is not fatal but please don't eat any of the foods below on a regular basis:

- Sugar, white or brown, and any syrup
- Honey, agave or any of its high-fructose corn syrup derivatives
- Artificial sweeteners
- Margarine
- Vegetable oils (including soybean, canola and rapeseed)
- Cereals that come in boxes (except plain oats)
- Diet drinks
- Energy drinks
- Fruit juices
- Crisps or rice cakes
- Baked delicacies including muffins, buns and other confectionery

Sugar or honey triggers weight gain and speeds up aging processes; they both contain high levels of fructose, which loads the liver and turns directly into fat. Do not eat foods that contain sugar in highly-available forms, such as sweets and white baked products. Never add sugar to your drinks and avoid drinks containing added sugars or sweeteners. Do not drink seemingly healthy fruit juices, which can often be higher in sugar than cool drinks. (You can follow this link to find out more about reading the sugar content from food labels: http://j.mp/1QmXStZ.)

Avoid processed oils like margarine and vegetable oils, which are made from fats that are highly reactive and promote inflammation. They can also have high trans-fat levels, which contribute to heart disease and increased cancer risks.

Try not to eat processed foods like bread, breakfast cereals, tinned foods, crisps and factory-made biscuits. Processed foods are low in nutrients, contain preservatives and colourants, and often have high sugar levels. Shun all fast-food whether made in fast-food restaurants or sold as ready-made meals. Also reduce your intake of processed meats like bacon, salami, ham, chicken nuggets and sausages.

Try at all times to keep the food you eat as close as possible to its original form.

These Banting No-Nos are now OK

You CAN eat these foods that were banned by Banting or low-carb:

- Rice (the best starch by far!)
- Potatoes, especially when served cold (because cold potato forms resistant starch, making a high percentage of the starch in the potato indigestible)
- Pasta and noodles (occasionally)
- Fruit, as long as it is in its natural form – avoid dried fruit, it is especially high in sugar. Fruit is high in fructose, which can harm your health in high doses. Fruits with lower fructose levels include berries and apples. Grapes have high fructose levels, as do bananas and oranges. Healthy fruits include olives, coconut, avocado and pawpaw.
- Bread in moderation. If you do eat bread, try to eat healthier varieties and avoid mass-produced supermarket types. Health breads that are gluten free, use coconut flour, sprouted grains and are made with butter are healthier choices.

There is no vegetable discrimination! Vegetables, including potatoes and sweet potatoes, are OK.

Fruit is fine. If it is part of a meal it is allowed, but it has to be in its original form. Real, whole fruit comes with its fibre and will not be harmful to you. However, when fruit is juiced, it is separated from its fibre and becomes much less healthy. Remember that fruit is high in fructose, which increases insulin resistance, so if you have a lot of weight to lose, don't eat a lot of fruit.

Pasta is also allowed occasionally but should be avoided if you are sensitive to gluten and wheat products, or if you suffer from any auto-immune condition. I would suggest that excess bread is avoided but see no harm in the occasional slice (or two) of bread once or twice a week, a toasted sandwich, or even a pizza every now and then.

Allowed foods

- All vegetables in their original form, raw or cooked
- Protein including meat, poultry and fish, but limit quantities to reasonable helpings. Always keep daily protein intake to around one gram of protein per kilogram of body weight
- Dairy of all kinds but limit milk if possible (milk is high in sugar and should preferably be replaced by cream, which has half the sugar and more fat). If you do drink milk, always drink it as full-fat and stay away from low or reduced fat milks as they often have added sugar to replace the loss of taste caused by the reduction of fat.
- Nuts, all kinds
- Alcohol: as part of a meal, all alcohol is allowed in moderation. Pure spirits are preferred when mixed with water or ice. A

glass of wine or a double tot of spirits like whiskey, brandy, gin or vodka daily with dinner is acceptable.

Eating rules

These are the non-negotiable rules for eating:
- **Eat bigger meals** less often (on any day, fasting or not)
- **Eat more fat**
- **No snacking** between meals (on any day, fasting or not)
- **Fast**, using a restricted eating window, one or more times a week

The general idea is to eat properly when you do eat. Accept that after a big meal, a large insulin spike will be produced but this big rise will be negated by a prolonged drop in insulin levels until the next big meal. This is why not snacking is so important; a nibble between meals causes an insulin ripple that raises average insulin levels and will prevent or delay restoration of insulin sensitivity.

Now, let's look at our rules in more detail.

Eat bigger meals

Remember that eating fewer meals is your goal, even on non-fasting days. Always, always eat until you are satisfied (but not uncomfortable) and then allow for a proper break between meals to give your insulin levels time to drop. Don't worry too much about quantities.

- One meal a day is allowed on fasting days (you can centre your fasting days around any meal; dinner is the most popular as it allows you to eat with family and friends, but some find lunch more convenient).

- On non-fasting days eat two or, at most, three normal meals.
- When you do eat, make it count; rather than have a small meal that will leave you hungry in a few hours, eat a bigger meal that will allow you to last longer before you have to eat again.

Eat more fat

In order to better balance your carb and protein consumption, it is necessary to increase the quantity of fat in your diet. Good healthy fat is good for you despite the last 50 years of medical propaganda demonising animal fats. Saturated (animal) fat does not cause high cholesterol or heart disease; this is, in fact, caused by high-sugar diets. Good healthy fats include avocados, cream, butter, lard, olive oil and egg yolks. Eating fatty portions of meat and chicken (with the skin) will contribute to a higher fat diet and will keep you fuller for longer after meals.

No snacking

Avoid snacking at all costs!

A snack between meals is dietary sabotage. Beware the tyranny of the quick, unconscious nibble driven by boredom more than need. Mindless grazing like this, swallowing without tasting, causes more damage than it's worth. All it takes is a small morsel or nibble between meals to sabotage your day.

Don't beat yourself up. Allow yourself an occasional lapse but be careful not to turn a small mistake into a habit that will wreck your diet.

Fast

The question is: how many times a week should you fast?

Initially, that depends on how much weight you need to lose. There are two cases when fasting more often brings better results:

- You have more than 10 kilograms to lose
- You have plateaued on Banting (or another diet)

Multiple days of fasting weekly will speed up weight loss. However, you may need some time to get used to not eating; teaching your body to handle periods of fasting takes some effort.

The best way to start is to use a strategy that moves breakfast later and later in the morning until it merges with your lunch (see the chapter Foundations of Fasting for more detailed instructions).

Some possible weekly fasting routines:

- Fast Tuesday and Thursday
- Fast Monday, Wednesday and Friday
- Fast Monday to Friday

All the above examples still allow you to 'go a little mad' over the weekend, as long as you stick to three meals per day and remember not to snack! Try them out and see what works for you. Sometimes you may find that you fast all day and are still not hungry by dinnertime. If this happens, then don't eat. The key is to listen to your body and to eat when you are hungry. This rule applies even when you are breaking a fast; sometimes you will be ravenously hungry (go ahead and eat as much as you need to) while other times you may find that you become full quickly. In either case, listen to your body and you will be fine.

Tricks and tips

Eating makes you hungry!

Many people find that as soon as they start to eat, they need to eat some more. My patients often tell me that once they start a day with eating breakfast, they remain hungry all day. What happens is that after a meal a cascade of hormones is released and some of these drive hunger.

Sometimes you will find that you become absolutely ravenous during a fast. When this happens, and you can't tough it out, don't give in and break the fast – try this tip instead: eat a high-fat food that does not stimulate insulin release. High-fat foods include butter (unsalted), plain avocado, or a tablespoon of coconut oil. This will make you feel full, but it's best to try the tough route and not use this option too often.

CHAPTER 15

THE NEW DEAL FOR DIABETICS

'My doctor told me to inject every morning when I wake up.'
Type 2 diabetic mantra

Warning: In all cases, this advice needs to be discussed with your doctor.

The New Deal will work well for type 2 diabetics, but it is not suitable for type 1 diabetics.

Type 1 diabetics

Type 1 diabetics do not make any insulin and they depend on injectable insulin for their survival. This means that type 1s are initially not insulin-resistant but insulin resistance can develop over time and being sedentary and overweight may predispose to it. Type 1 diabetics cannot follow the New Deal, which is designed to lower insulin levels and reduce insulin resistance.

Type 1s need to be aware of the dangers of insulin and that lowering the units of insulin that they inject daily is still desirable. Periods of fasting are still beneficial for type 1s, as long as blood sugar levels are carefully monitored and care is taken to stay well hydrated. A 2007 study of prolonged fasting in type 1s, published in the *Diabetic Medicine Journal*, reported 'Persons with type 1 diabetes can participate safely in prolonged fasts provided they reduce their usual insulin dose significantly and adhere to guidelines regarding glucose monitoring and indications for terminating fasting'. In addition, the benefits of low carb principles and increased exercise need to be explored within the context of each type 1 diabetic's management and in conjunction with their doctor's advice.

Type 2 diabetics

An initial diagnosis of type 2 diabetes puts most patients on a fixed path of steadily increasing diabetic medications. Most patients are started on a single tablet that is designed to increase their production of insulin. Thereafter, there is a steady progression of higher doses that are often then followed by either additional oral medicine or insulin injections, or in some cases, both. Current medical therapy offers no cure; treatment strategy is based on steadily increasing medications until the patient finally dies, closely resembling a treadmill that slowly increases speed until the patient falls off. The more insulin the patient takes, the more their insulin resistance increases and thus the more insulin that is required. Prolonged high insulin levels are not good for anyone and have profound health implications. (If you need a reminder of these, read the chapter Know your enemy, its name is Insulin.)

Taking more insulin increases insulin resistance, which is what caused the type 2 diabetes in the first place. We end up treating a disease of too much insulin with more insulin.

Decreasing insulin resistance and reducing insulin requirements is a far better strategy for treating type 2 diabetes. This can be accomplished with dietary and lifestyle changes.

Strategies for dealing with type 2 diabetes

Low-carb: The first step is to follow a low-carb diet. The basic Banting diet or a low-carb diet as described in my book, *The Decarb Diet,* is ideal for lowering insulin or diabetic medication requirements. As carbohydrate intake is reduced, blood sugar levels come down, reducing the need for diabetic medication. Low-carb regimens can be improved even further with reductions in daily protein intake to levels of 1 gram of protein per kilogram of body weight, or even slightly less.

Exercise: Being sedentary, sitting for long periods, and avoiding exercise increases insulin resistance, often adding to weight-gain tendencies. Despite the lack of energy that often accompanies type 2 diabetes, some form of exercise always helps. Sitting less and walking more is a good place to start. For any type of exercise, I recommend shorter bursts of activity at higher exertion levels rather than long, slow efforts. An hour of slow walking on a treadmill can easily be shortened to a 20-minute session of interval training which has a better effect on insulin sensitivity and frees up more time. For more information on exercising, read the chapter Move further on in this book.

Intermittent fasting

Fasting a few days a week will reduce diabetic medication requirements even further. The effects are felt on two levels: eating less food reduces insulin requirements, and periods without food result in increased insulin sensitivity, which means that less insulin is required to produce the same results.

Eating less can cure type 2 diabetes. One drastic way to eat less is to have bariatric surgery. As so eloquently explained by Dr Jason

Fung in his video 'The two big lies of type 2 diabetes' (http://j. mp/1L0BJoy), type 2 diabetes can be cured by surgery where the stomach is stapled, producing a state of enforced fasting. This cures type 2 diabetes in almost all patients for at least two to three years after the operation.

The same result can be achieved in a much easier way with intermittent fasting. However, this does require a change of mindset because a common recommendation is to inject insulin or to take diabetic medication as soon as you wake up in the morning. This seems to make sense because blood sugar levels are often raised when one wakes up. However, taking medication, especially injecting with insulin, immediately requires that some food be consumed for the insulin to act on.

A better strategy is not to eat breakfast and not to inject with insulin, while carefully monitoring blood sugar levels. Generally, blood sugar levels will not increase without the consumption of food and will usually drop or stabilise during the course of the morning.

My suggestion is to start by skipping breakfast and then gradually push the fasting window to lunchtime and then to dinnertime. You can use the recommendation for fasting given in the chapter Foundations of fasting.

Blood sugar levels need to be carefully monitored at all times. If blood sugar levels drop too low, eat a small meal to prevent a sugar low. Be aware that medication requirements will be reduced! If you have any doubts ask your doctor for help.

In the video, 'The two big lies of type 2 diabetes' (http://j. mp/1L0BJoy) you can listen to the testimonials of two of Dr Jason Fung's patients who used fasting to come off their medications and lose weight at the same time. One of these patients started off by fasting and drinking only unsweetened fluids for three weeks, without any ill effects.

CHAPTER 16

EATING REAL

'Real food does not have ingredients,
real food is ingredients.'
Jamie Oliver

The beaches of Brittany in France are home to some of nature's most spectacular seascapes. Perfect beaches with crashing breakers, teeming rock pools and sandy expanses framed by verdant greenery make them ideal destinations for a holiday by the sea. It was on one of these beaches, called Saint-Michel-en-Grève, that Vincent Petit, a young veterinarian, galloped across on his horse in August 2009, both of them revelling in the thrill of the ride over the sands. Their joy was short-lived, ending in disaster, when they slipped into a pool of decomposing algae that released toxic gasses that quickly took the horse's life and rendered Petit unconscious. Fortunately, his life was saved by passers-by who dragged him out of the stinking morass.

Not so coincidentally, Brittany is also home to more than half the pigs in France. Enough pigs to produce 415,000 tons of meat in 2012, according to a publication *The Pig Industry in Brittany* (2013). The rivers of pig poo that these pigs produce are disposed of in desperation as a slurry that is spread over the crop fields of Brittany. Rain, when it falls, leaches large quantities of phosphates and nitrogen from this slurry into the water that eventually drains into the sea. The local seawater, swollen with unnaturally high levels of these nutrients, becomes an ideal medium for algae to grow in. These algae, called sea lettuce, grow in massive banks that deplete the sea around them of oxygen, causing the death of fish and other sea fauna. Pieces of algae break off and wash up onto the beach, forming large rotting masses, similar to the one that claimed the life of Petit's horse.

The machinations of the messy, stinky business that produces the food we eat is a million miles away from the clean aisles of our modern supermarkets, which belie the often horrific origins of the stuff that ends up in our trolleys. Mass production methods, designed to eke every last drop of value from concentrated feeding operations, pay our health and the wellbeing of the environment little heed. The consequences of some of the methods they employ are only just becoming evident. Antibiotic consumption by the meat and poultry we consume exceeds 50% of total world production, which is leading to the development of superbugs that threaten to render most of our antibiotics useless.

Vegetarian readers may feel somewhat insulated from the kind of barbarity that meat eaters ignore or know little about. However, the agricultural industry that grows vegetarian food is little better. Certain modern crops are genetically engineered to be resistant to pesticides to the extent that some seeds for growing crops are paired with pesticides that the seeds have been engineered to be resistant to. This allows farmers to use massive doses of toxic concoctions that kill anything growing except the crops.

On a recent mountain bike ride in the Maluti mountain area of South Africa, some friends and I rode through breathtaking vistas reminiscent of Van Gogh's wheat fields and came across a group of farm workers mixing pesticides for crop spraying. Fumes from their potion hung heavy in the air and we struggled for breath as the noisome miasma threatened to sear our lungs. Yet as unlikely as it seems, pesticide manufacturers claim that these kinds of fertilisers are harmless to humans. This may be true, but in the meantime we, the consumers, are turned unwittingly into lab rats who may only know the truth many years from now.

I am well aware that most of us have little option other than to eat the meat produced by Concentrated Animal Feeding Operations (CAFO) as well as the genetically-modified (GMO) agricultural products that line our shelves. However, armed with a little knowledge, we still have options available to us to limit our exposure.

Over and above any pesticide, antibiotic or hormone residues, our bodies also face the challenge of digesting food containing reduced levels of minerals, antioxidants and vital omega-3 fatty acids. On top of this, our food supply is saturated with sugar and corn sugar (HFCS) derivatives, which are added to almost every type of processed food.

The missing Omega-3s

Any discussion about real food has to include the critical omega-3 fats, which are presently all but absent from our modern food supply. Our cell membranes (walls) are built from omega-3 and omega-6 fatty acids and a disturbance in the ratio of these fats affects the structural integrity of the cell walls, causing them to leak. It is believed that some cancers, as well as atherosclerosis of the arteries, are caused by this kind of damage.

It has been estimated that in ancestral times, our food supply had an omega-3 to omega-6 ratio of 1:1. In those times, the food chain began with creatures who ate green foliage or algae, which en-masse represents the largest source of fats on the planet in the form of alpha-linolenic acid (ALA). Further on up the food chain, leaf or algae-eating creatures were themselves eaten by carnivorous animals, who then incorporated these fats into their tissues (usually in the form of EPA and DHA). Modern farming methods have broken this ancient food chain and now feed our food chain predominantly with omega-6-rich grains.

The result is that our food supply today has an omega-3 to omega-6 ratio of about 1:20, heavily skewed in favour of the inflammatory omega-6s. The economics behind this are simple; omega-3s and shelf-life are mutually exclusive and the higher the omega-3 content of a foodstuff, the faster it goes off. As a result, the omega-3s in almost all the food in our supermarkets have been removed to make products last longer.

One of the processes food manufacturers use to promote shelf-life is to hydrogenate omega-3 fatty acids, which turns good fats into bad trans-fats. Foods that have been processed in this way carry the seemingly inoffensive terms 'partially hydrogenated' or 'hydrogenated' on their ingredients labels. Look out for these words on the food you buy and do not eat them if you value your health.

Remember the story about the guy who found a perfectly preserved burger in his coat pocket 14 years after he bought it? It still looked the same as it did when he bought it because it contained no omega-3s.

Eating real food

Eating real, natural food takes a little more time and energy, as well as some knowledge about what 'real' and 'natural' mean. Trying to fill your trolley, keeping costs low and still buying 'real' as you walk the aisles of a modern supermarket is a challenge. Shelves are heavy with processed foods and any original grown produce may be basted in pesticides and thawing out from months of hibernation in a deep freeze.

Unfortunately, there is no 'How to eat real food 101' course that you can sign up for. In the following sections, I present an overview of what to look for and what to avoid when trying to eat real food. Nowadays you need to be a well-informed hunter-gatherer to feed yourself and your family in the safest, least harmful way.

In addition to the eating of natural foods, I also cover areas relating to common daily-use chemicals, as well as some critical details about the gut and how it affects your health.

Basic guidelines

Eat natural food as often as you can. Natural food is easy to recognise as it does not normally come in boxes, is never advertised on TV, and seldom comes with a 'Nutrition facts' label. Ready-made meals, instant foods and food bought from fast food and take-away joints are usually as far as you can get from real or natural. Eating vegetables and fruits that are preferably organically grown is a good place to start.

What you drink is also important. Keep it clean with fresh, filtered water and avoid all sodas, energy drinks and sweetened concoctions. Water is often sold in flavoured form, which in many instances has added sugar, sweeteners or preservatives, and should therefore be avoided. Sparkling water is fine to drink as long as it is not mixed with any additives.

Here is a summary of the general guidelines, each of which is explained in more detail in the sections below.

Water

- Install a good water filter in your home
- Drink filtered water whenever possible
- Never use water from the hot water tap for drinking or cooking
- Never drink water bottled in plastic containers, unless you have no choice (the plasticizers used to make low-cost bottles are hormone disruptors that dissolve into the water)
- Use a glass water bottle for carrying water around in and for drinking in the gym

Meat

- Eat little or no processed, cured, smoked meat (processed meats contain nitrites that are known to promote cancer)
- Try to eat grass-fed or organic meat when possible
- Eat fatty meat in preference to lean cuts
- Don't eat more than 200 grams of meat on any single day

Poultry (applies to turkey as well)

- Eat organic chicken and eggs when possible
- Eat free-range when organic is not available
- Eat chicken with the skin to increase fat content relative to protein

- Do not consume large quantities of 'white' chicken meat without balancing this high protein intake with a similar amount of fat like butter, olive oil or avocado.

Poultry – eggs

- Eat whole eggs; yolks contain almost all the beneficial nutrients and minerals
- Eggs will not raise your cholesterol
- Buy organic eggs when possible
- Avoid eggs with pale yolks; the deeper the yolk's yellow, the higher its omega-3 content
- Eggs are best eaten as close to raw as possible; heat them as little as you can tolerate, because the extra heat oxidises the cholesterol, which then becomes a trigger for inflammation
- Soft-boiled eggs are a good compromise; cool your boiled eggs down immediately after cooking to limit further heat damage

Fish

- Eat less tuna, mackerel, swordfish and other large fish because they have higher heavy metal levels than small fish like pilchards and herrings
- Avoid tinned fish (the tins are lined with plastic, from which plasticizers are leached into the fish meat)
- Eat wild-caught fish when possible
- Avoid farmed salmon; it has high levels of a synthetic petro-chemical based additive that is used to give it a pink colour
- Combining leafy green vegetables with your fish meal can help to reduce heavy metal absorption; chlorella supplements can also help

- A good source of information about good fish selection is the Seafood Selector website of the Environmental Defense Fund (http://seafood.edf.org)

Sugar and fructose

- Avoid eating or drinking foods that have a high sugar content; in addition to the diabetes risks, high blood sugar levels make you age faster
- Sugar is 50% fructose, which worsens insulin resistance and leads to a fatty liver; fructose is treated the same way as alcohol by the body
- Sugar increases uric acid
- Honey is not a health food! It is sugar in a liquid form
- Agave is not a health food. Avoid it at all costs; it has higher fructose levels than honey

Artificial sweeteners

- Avoid all artificial sweeteners and drinks containing them, especially cold drinks
- Artificial sweeteners cause weight gain by raising insulin levels as much as sugar does
- Splenda (Sucralose) has just been downgraded to 'Avoid' rather than 'Caution' because of increased cancer risks
- Artificial sweeteners damage your gut and encourage the growth of bad gut bacteria
- They make you fatter and more hungry
- If you do use an artificial sweetener, consider stevia, which has no nutritive value, or else use xylitol

Sports and energy drinks

- Sports and energy drinks contain high sugar levels for no real reason
- They dissolve your teeth
- Energy drinks have high caffeine levels as well as other chemical supplements that can lead to health problems

Cereal grains

Corn

- Don't eat corn or corn-based products (80% or more of South African corn is GMO and despite assurances of the complete safety of GMO foods by governments and companies like Monsanto, an internet search will quickly reveal how many authorities disagree)
- Don't eat products that contain high fructose corn syrup (HFCS)

Wheat

- Eat sparingly; sugar makes up 50% or more of most wheat products
- The gluten in wheat can have subtle but damaging effects on the health of people who are sensitive to it. Symptoms can include general tiredness, bloating, irritability, joint pain and headaches
- All auto-immune disease sufferers should eat a strictly gluten-free diet for at least three to six months in order to ascertain how much their symptoms are affected by gluten consumption

Rice

- Rice is the best starch choice
- It is the least genetically modified grain
- If you are avoiding gluten, eat sticky rice as it contains no gluten

Dairy

- Milk should be avoided or consumed in limited quantities. For example, by swapping cappuccinos for long blacks (Americanos) with pouring cream, you can reduce milk intake by 80% per cup, which greatly reduces the quantity of milk you consume. The cream has more fat and will keep you full for longer
- A tablespoon of cream in black coffee during fasting days is perfect for improving the taste and will have minimal impact on insulin levels
- Drink A2 milk when you are in countries that offer this variety (South African milk is A2; the A1 variety has a protein structure that can cause allergic effects)
- Butter is the best food you can feed your gut. It contains butyrate which is the primary food of many beneficial large gut bacteria. Always use it for cooking; never use margarine or any other vegetable oils. Avoid all oils, cooking or food products that have the word 'hydrogenated' on their labels

Alcohol

The New Deal specifically allows for the careful consumption of alcohol, which means following these basic rules:
- Always drink alcohol in moderation
- Drink alcohol at most 3 or 4 times a week

- Mix drinks with water or ice only
- To reduce sugar intake, avoid cocktails and fruit-based drinks
- If you are trying to eat gluten free, avoid grain-based alcohols

Soy

- Say NO to soy and soy products *except* fermented soy products like miso, natto, tempeh, and others
- Soy has estrogen-like effects and can alter menstrual cycles and promote breast cancer
- These estrogen-like effects also promote weight retention and gain
- Never ever give soy milk to infants; it will speed up their sexual development

Coffee

- Drink filtered coffee in preference to instant coffee
- Avoid decaf coffee if you can as it may still contain residues of the chemicals used to make it
- Limit coffee intake to no more than three or four cups a day

Probiotics

Probiotics are live bacteria as yeasts that contribute the 'good' flora in your gut.

- Regularly eat fresh fermented foods like sauerkraut and pickled foodstuffs (they contain large colonies of live beneficial bacteria)
- Take a probiotic supplement from time to time; usually the more expensive varieties are a better investment

- Consider making your own fermented foods; sauerkraut is easy to make and requires no more than some cabbage and seasoning
- Growing and eating your own vegetables is a good way to consume live probiotics (don't over wash them)

Daily-use items to avoid

- Commercial table salt (it has a reduced mineral content and contains chemicals that allow it to flow easily and prevent clumping); use Himalayan pink salt instead
- Water or food in plastic containers
- Anti-bacterial soaps, dishwashing liquids and detergents (they contain chemicals that are absorbed into the skin and needlessly kill bacteria that cause us no harm)
- Tinned foods
- Toothpaste – use as little as possible and never swallow it (it contains chemicals that are bad for your gut)
- Mouthwash (as above)

Detailed guidelines

Water

Drink filtered water whenever you can. In 2009, the Environmental Working Group in the USA reported that they had found over 300 pollutants contaminating drinking water, half of which were not yet subject to health regulation but which you can be sure have no place in a healthy body.

The most important place to start is by fitting a water filter in your home. There are many options available ranging from simple filter jugs to elaborate reverse osmosis systems that need to be installed below your kitchen sick. Choosing a more effective system can be expensive but could protect you from many future health issues. Another route of toxic contamination from your home water supply is from bath or shower water and some experts suggest that this water should also be filtered. Contaminants are absorbed into the skin during bathing; the hotter the water, the more easily they are absorbed. Despite government regulations or public announcements about how pure our drinking water is, there is no way to control how our water is delivered. Clean processed water has a long way to go before it gushes out of your tap and can be contaminated in many ways. It can be exposed to external pollutants or it may come into contact with myriad toxic materials in the network of pipes it passes through on its way to you.

There is strong medical evidence implicating unfiltered tap water as a probable cause of disease. A 2005 report in the *International Journal of Cancer* found that men drinking tap water had an almost 50% increased risk of developing bladder cancer compared to men who drank filtered water. The study suggested that the higher risk was caused by carcinogenic chemicals present in tap water.

To protect yourself and your family, you can apply some general safety rules:

Don't drink or cook with water from a hot water tap. It is surprising how many people fill their kettles from the hot water tap, perhaps thinking that it will save time boiling their kettles. The minimal time and energy saved comes with significantly increased health risks. Hot water does a much better job of leaching metals like lead and copper from the pipes it runs through. In addition, hot water geysers accumulate sludge that can slowly contaminate the water they heat.

When drinking unfiltered tap water: If possible, run the tap for 20 or 30 seconds to clear any water that has been standing in the pipes to ensure that you drink the cleanest, freshest water possible.

Plastic bottled water: Don't regularly drink water in plastic bottles. Never re-use old plastic drinking bottles; they are made of cheap plastic that leaches toxic chemicals like bisphenol A (BPA) into your drink. BPA is a feminising hormone that can wreak hormonal havoc in your body. (See the section below 'Plastic bottles and containers' in 'Daily-use items to avoid' for more info.) If you are one of those people who habitually carries drinking water around with you, do your health a favour and get yourself a good quality glass bottle. Be especially wary of drinking from a warm plastic bottle; never take a plastic water bottle into the sauna and never leave plastic water bottles in your car as they can give off toxic chemicals when heated by the sun.

Meat

Avoid manufactured or processed meat products that are cured, smoked, salted or have preservatives added. These kinds of meats include sausages, bacon, ham and salami. Many studies have connected the eating of these types of meats with an increased risk of developing high blood pressure, as well as bowl, stomach, pancreatic and bladder cancer. Various agents are added to processed meats, such as nitrite and nitrosamines, to enhance the pink colour and to prevent the fat in the meat from going rancid.

If you do buy processed meats, try to ensure that they are 100% meat and do not contain added 'padding' in the form of vegetable or other matter.

There are three types of meat classifications to be aware of (in order of preference):

- Grass-fed
- Grain-finished
- Grain-fed

Always go for **grass-fed** meat if you can afford to pay the extra cost; the best place to buy grass-fed is at smaller, specialty butcher shops. This kind of beef tastes better and, if you look carefully, has fat that is a little yellow in colour. The yellow comes from the increased omega-3 content because the cattle have grazed on green, fresh grass. Grass-fed meat also has higher CLA levels (Conjugated Linoleic Acid), which is anecdotally linked to body leanness and anti-cancer properties.

Grain-finished represents the middle ground between grass and grain-fed. Grain-finished cattle start out eating grass and are then 'finished' with grain in the last weeks of their lives. The grain bulks them up and fattens them, allowing the farmer to deliver more meat to market.

Grain-fed cattle are normally raised in confined feed-lots where they eat grain- or soy-based feed that is often laced with chemicals to reduce infections and to increase the size of the animals. This process results in high omega-6 levels, with a large reduction in omega-3 and CLA content.

Eat fattier portions: Whether you are following a low-carb diet or not, be mindful of the quantity of protein a lean portion of meat actually contains. Limit your daily protein consumption to about one gram of protein per kilogram of body weight. (See the chapter *Excess protein – Banting's major weakness* for more information about the danger of protein over consumption.) When you can, eat fattier meat portions that reduce your overall protein intake.

Poultry

Chicken has become increasingly popular and has overtaken beef as the animal protein of choice in many countries. This is driven by a number of factors including lower prices as well as nutritional guidelines that suggest chicken meat as a 'healthy', low-fat alternative to beef. Because most non-vegetarians eat chicken a few times a week, it is a good idea to have some background information about how our chicken is made.

Commercial chickens are reared for market indoors. This includes the production of chicken eggs, which are laid in massive sheds by thousands of hens. Their beaks are severed by lasers to prevent them from pecking each other, which happens often as each animal has a space the size of an A4 sheet of paper in which to live. Hens like these will never see the sun, nor will they walk on grass or peck the ground in search of the grubs that are part of their staple diet. Instead, they eat corn or soy under artificial lights and after laying eggs for 70 weeks, they are slaughtered to make way for a fresh batch of laying hens.

In confined chicken breeding operations like these, chickens are usually fed antibiotics, which often contain arsenic that can still be detectable at supermarket level. In 2014, the U.S. Food and Drug Administration (FDA) reported that up to 70% of chicken on the shelves in supermarkets contained detectable quantities of arsenic. This should be of interest to South African chicken eaters; according to the South African Revenue Services, 457,374 tons of chicken were imported into South Africa during 2015.

Bacterial contamination of chicken meat, usually with Salmonella, is also common and the USDA Food Safety and Inspection Service reports that each year about 150,000 Americans contract stomach disorders from eating contaminated meat.

Where feasible, the solution is not to buy chicken that comes from large supermarket chains and to preferably source chicken that is reared by smaller local farming operations. Organic chickens from smaller farms live a more natural life and spend their days outside eating a mixture of greenery and insects, producing yolks with high omega-3 content. Their diet can also be supplemented with grain-based feed that does not contain hormones or antibiotics.

(Note: When buying chicken, any 'grade' information that may appear on the label refers to a physical assessment of the look of the chicken, which takes fat content and bone structure into account and has nothing to do with how the animal was raised.)

Housing

- **Organic**: reared with full access to normal outdoor farm conditions

- **Free-range**: chickens have some access to roam and feed outdoors (some manufacturers use this label for chickens that have extremely limited outdoor access, since the term has no legal definition)

- **Pastured**: similar to free-range but in general more likely to have had proper outdoor access

Eggs

The colour of the yolk is a good indication of the omega-3 content; a brighter yellow colour signifies higher levels of omega-3s. Pale yolks are produced by grain-based feed and are high in omega-6 fatty acids with no appreciable levels of omega-3s.

Fish

Although fish is often seen as a healthy alternative protein source to meat and poultry, there are some concerns around increased fish consumption.

Heavy metal contamination: The concentration of heavy metals like mercury, lead and cadmium vary widely depending on where the fish was caught, as well as the size of the fish. Larger fish that have lived longer accumulate more heavy metals because of their age and the fact that they consume other fish, which magnifies the levels of heavy metals they consume. Because of this, shark, tuna, mackerel and swordfish have the highest levels of heavy metals. Herrings, for example, are small fish and normally have mercury levels that are ten times lower than those of shark or tuna.

Fish farming: Aquaculture produces about 50% of the fish consumed in the world. While this may sound like a good way to reduce the risks of over-fishing, confined fishing operations produce inferior fish. One of the big draw cards of fish consumption is the high omega-3 levels they contain, but factory-farmed fish usually have low levels because, when possible, they are fed a grain-based diet. Dr Anne-Lise Birch Monsen of the University of Bergen, Norway, caused a stir in 2013 when she raised concerns about the increased levels of toxic contaminants in farmed salmon. One of these contaminants is synthetic astaxanthin, which is fed to the farmed salmon to turn their flesh pink since they naturally have grey-coloured flesh, which is not acceptable to consumers. Synthetic astaxanthin has never been tested or approved for human consumption and must not be confused with the natural form, which is sold as a potent anti-oxidant supplement.

Sugar and fructose

As I've mention elsewhere, sugar in highly available form should not be part of any healthy, natural diet. Today it is becoming fashionable to be anti-sugar, which is great news because sugar has many health drawbacks:

- Sugar is made of equal parts of glucose and fructose. Once digested, the fructose half of sugar can only be dealt with in the liver where it is converted into triglycerides, a form of fat. The uric acid produced as a waste product of this conversion can lead to gout as well as high blood pressure. It does this by suppressing nitric oxide levels in the walls of blood vessels causing them to constrict more, thus raising blood pressure.

- The triglycerides from the converted fructose are then stored in the liver as fat droplets. If enough of these fat droplets accumulate, the liver becomes enlarged and sometimes inflamed, resulting in fatty liver disease. Not to be confused with the alcohol-produced variety, NAFLD (Non-Alcoholic Fatty Liver Disease) occurs in people who consume too much sugar. It is the most common disease in children in the USA today, affecting one in every ten children.

- Another problem with the consumption of sugar is that it seems to bypass our built-in 'fullness' sensors. Various studies have shown that sweet drinks added to a meal have no effect on this sensation, which means that you still eat the same quantity at a session irrespective of whether you drink soda or water.

Honey: This widely renowned 'health food' is nothing of the kind. While it is possible that honey contains some bee proteins that are healthy, the fact remains that honey is liquid sugar. High fructose corn syrup (HFCS), which is produced chemically from corn, is so similar to honey that only lab tests can differentiate them. The effects of honey are also the same as sugar; increased insulin resistance, inflammation, raised blood pressure and weight gain. This was recently confirmed by a 2015 *Journal of Nutrition* study that compared the effects of honey, sugar and HFCS and found their ill-effects to be identical.

Agave: This sugar substitute is higher in fructose than honey or HFCS. Fructose content as high as 75% is not unusual; this 'health' food is often manufactured from HCFS, despite its claimed natural origins.

By adhering to the list under 'Foods to be avoided' in the chapter *A new deal*, you will be able to avoid most forms of concentrated sugars in your diet. You can also learn how to read the nutrition facts labels that appear on the packaging of most processed food items (visit DrRybko.com: http://j.mp/1QmXStZ for more information). This will help you to identify foods that, despite their appearance, have high sugar content.

Artificial sweeteners

From a weight loss perspective it is well documented by several large studies that artificial sweeteners cause weight gain. The reason for this is our old friend insulin. It has now become clear that artificial sweeteners, like aspartame, raise insulin levels as high as sugar does. Any diet aimed at keeping insulin levels low will fail when faced with regular intake of these man-made sugar substitutes.

To help scare you off, below are the five artificial sweeteners approved by the FDA, all of which have received health warnings from various quarters:

- *Saccharin*: implicated in bladder cancer

- *Acesulfame-K*: may contain methylene chloride residue and cause mental issues such as headaches and mood swings. Also implicated in cancer, liver and kidney disease

- *Aspartame (NutraSweet, Equal)*: increased risk of leukemia and lymphoma in rats and also linked as a possible cause of these diseases in a 2012 American Society for Nutrition study

- *Neotame*: a relatively new addition that is based on aspartame, designed to remove the requirement of aspartame to carry a health warning for phenylketonuria (an inherited inability to metabolize phenylalanine which, if untreated, causes brain and nerve damage)

- *Sucralose*: labelled as 'Avoid' in 2016 by the Center for Science in the Public Interest because of a new animal study that indicates it poses a cancer risk

In summary, avoid all sweeteners! If you feel that you really need to use an agent to replace the sugar in your food, consider stevia, which is a natural sweetener, or otherwise xylitol, which does have some caloric value but is safe to use in moderation.

Sports and energy drinks

Just say no to these; rather drink water! I can see no reason why anyone would drink one of the many sports drinks on the market, such as Energade and Powerade, and would say the same thing about energy drinks, the most famous of which is Red Bull. Obviously, consumers don't agree with me and the energy drink market brought in over $10 billion in 2012 in the U.S. alone.

Sports drinks: These kinds of drinks are marketed at just about anyone who exercises and can often be seen clutched in the hands of earnest shoppers darting around in the mall. Besides the fact that they contain high quantities of largely unnecessary carbohydrates in various guises, they have other downsides as well. One of these is the effect that sports drinks have on your teeth. Because most of the drinks are acidic in order to prolong shelf-life, they can literally eat your teeth away. A recent study at Birmingham University in the UK showed that when a sports drink has a relatively high pH and low calcium content, it would have high erosive potential on tooth enamel.

Cost is another issue. Why pay so much for these kinds of drinks if plain water would do? In addition, these drinks may have high salt levels (sodium and potassium), which lead to increased thirst.

Energy drinks: Energy drinks are worse for you than sports drinks for two main reasons. First, they contain added caffeine that gets delivered in a single jolt (unlike the way a coffee is sipped). This shot of caffeine is the reason why energy drinks can be marketed as 'speed in a can'; they deliver a shock strong enough to resurrect a dead horse. Second, they are usually taken outside the exercise environment and, as a result, produce a sugar rush that, in the absence of muscular exertion, has nowhere to go except to fat stores. Energy drinks can also contain herbal supplements, taurine and other chemicals that have not been properly tested in medical trials. There are numerous reports in medical literature about the dangers of consuming energy drinks. Medical consequences include seizures, cardiac emergencies and abnormalities, mood alterations and diabetes. Children and young adults seem to be especially at risk.

Cereal grains

Edible grasses such as maize (corn), wheat and rice provide by far the greatest portion of the world's food supply. Grains have only been domesticated for use as food in the last 10,000 years. In evolutionary terms, this is the blink of an eye and as a result, not all humans have properly adapted to eating them.

In the last 100 years, genetic manipulation of these grains has proceeded in two directions. Initially, by genetic manipulation within the grass species. This produced production-friendly crops like American biologist Norman Borluag's dwarf wheat, which greatly increased yields and has fed millions at the expense of exposing us to many new antigens and proteins. More recently, and much more frighteningly, genetic manipulation has been performed between species. Here, bacterial genes, for example, are spliced into the genes of food-producing plants to produce something new, a genetically modified organism (GMO).

In the USA, these new GMOs are legally patentable, allowing companies like Monsanto to patent and hold legal rights to the seeds they sell. They exercised this right when they sued Percy Schmeiser, a Canadian canola farmer, for illegally growing their seeds. Schmeiser, who had never purchased Monsanto canola seeds, claimed that his crops had been contaminated from neighbouring farms. He refused Monsanto's request to pay licensing fees and as a result, they sued him successfully for planting their seeds without a license. This was a widely unpopular decision but it was upheld by the Canadian legal system all the way to the Canadian Supreme Court.

Corn

Corn is the world's largest grain crop and most of it is genetically modified, usually in one of two ways (and often in both). First, corn is altered to be 'herbicide resistant' so that it can tolerate higher levels of pesticide. This allows farmers to use higher concentrations of weed killers without harming the crop, which unfortunately translates into higher concentrations of these poisonous chemicals eventually ending up on our plates. In South Africa, glyphosate (Roundup) is extensively used in conjunction with glyphosate-resistant corn.

Second, the corn is designed to produce insecticides, which sounds like a fantasy from a high school science project, but actually happens. In 2015, Bt-corn, which has been genetically engineered so that every cell produces its own pesticide against the borer caterpillar, was planted on 81% of all American crop acres, thus delivering the fruits of pesticide-producing corn to the plates of millions of Americans (according to the U.S. Department of Agriculture).

How a rational civilisation could allow agri-business to graft bacteria genes into an edible plant defies all logic. However, like it or not, our largest food source now incorporates the DNA of a bacterium (Bacillus thuringiensis), and produces a natural pesticide in the form of crystal proteins that has unknown effects on us and the environment.

To me it's simple: if you want to eat a healthy diet, corn or corn products cannot be a part of the food you eat.

Wheat

While we are on the topic of sugar, it is important to realise that in some ways, wheat is sugar! Many of my patients firmly believe they avoid all forms of sugar. They then look horrified when I explain that bread and pasta, which are made from wheat, are between 50% and 70% sugar. During digestion, the sugars in wheat are rapidly absorbed, resulting in large blood sugar spikes and thus large insulin spikes.

Besides being high in sugars, wheat also contains an array of foreign substances, of which gluten is the most well-known. Although the New Deal allows for the eating of some bread and pasta, if you need to avoid gluten, do not eat these food items.

Gluten is widespread along our food supply. As well as occurring in obvious places such as wheat-containing products, it can pop up in unexpected places. Some brands of instant coffee and flavoured coffees, for example, contain some gluten. Be wary too of any food that says something like 'Gluten free but made in a factory that produces products containing gluten'. These kinds of foods often test positive for containing gluten, frequently in surprisingly high concentrations.

Gluten is just one of a number of foreign particles (antigens) that are incorporated into our food and produce an immune response in the gut. In an allergic person, gluten causes cell damage or death to cells in the gut wall. This leads to leaky gut and its associated auto-immune issues. Many studies suggest that gluten sensitivity is much more prevalent than is generally acknowledged.

Beware of gluten sensitivity, the effects of which often become so much a part of you that you incorporate these ill-effects into what you are, never realising how much better you would actually feel if it was removed from your diet. I can say with absolute confidence that if you suffer from any kind of auto-immune disease, such as eczema or skin conditions, arthritis or thyroid disease, you should eat gluten-free for at least three months to see how its absence affects you. In addition to an auto-immune disease, here are some of the signs that you may suffer from gluten sensitivity:

- Poor digestion (gas, bloating, constipation, diarrhea)
- Headaches after eating
- Depression
- Anxiety or irritability
- Difficulty in focusing
- Brain fog
- Joint pain
- General tiredness

Besides the issues above, wheat has been implicated (not proven) in certain nervous disorders like schizophrenia and autism. There have also been some medical studies that show unfavourable cholesterol changes (smaller LDL particle size) resulting from wheat consumption.

Dairy

Some people simply can't tolerate dairy, others may have a subtle allergy to it, but used carefully dairy can be a versatile and tasty addition to a real food diet.

No milk: I advise against drinking milk in any quantity and suggest that you avoid it as far as possible. Commercially available milk is subject to the worst kind of production excesses and as a result, it can become a potent anti-health food. It starts with milk-producing cows who are fed grains and soy-based foods, often laced with chemicals, instead of the green grass they are born to eat. In the USA and many other countries, the use of growth hormone (Bovine Somatotropin) to increase milk yields is legal. Then, the milk is pasteurised, a process that destroys crucial enzymes and bacteria.

Cream and butter are better. Substituting milk with cream in coffee reduces the lactose (milk sugar) content, while upping the fat content. Butter is good for you and for your gut. Many makes of grass-fed butter are available; the no-salt variety tastes so good that it can (and should) be eaten by the teaspoonful. This kind of butter is also ideal for making Bulletproof (butter- and coconut oil-based) coffee. Cheese is also okay but be careful not to eat it in large quantities, as it can be hard on the digestive system. Go for the older, matured varieties if you can.

Note: Most people who are lactose intolerant already know it. Here are some signs that you are dairy sensitive. After eating dairy food you:

- Have bloating and distension
- Have stomach cramps

- Can hear gas moving in your stomach
- Develop a runny tummy, usually with diarrhea

Besides lactose intolerance, some people also suffer from intolerance to casein, the main protein in milk. Casein comes in two varieties, A1 and A2. Some 10,000 years ago there was a split in the line of cows, resulting in cows that produce milk containing A1 casein, while others produce milk with the A2 variety. In some countries A2 milk is available and you should preferably buy this variety whenever you have the choice. All African cows produce A2 casein.

Say No to soy

Soy, in anything other than its fermented non-GMO form, is good for your health in the same way that smoking is good for your lungs. It is best to avoid all soy products such as:

- Soy milk
- Soy sauce
- Soy protein
- Tofu

Fermented soy products like tempeh, pickled tofu, natto and soy miso are okay, as long as they are non-GMO. Otherwise, try not to be swayed by the marketing campaigns of the soy manufacturers, a good example of which is the Consumer Attitudes About Nutrition report by the United Soybean Board, which shows that 75% of U.S. consumers rate soy products as healthy.

If you want to preserve or promote your gut health, consider that as much as 90% of the soy produced in the U.S. today is genetically modified (GMO) and, as a result, contains the highest possible pesticide levels, usually glyphosate, which are toxic to the gut.

Other possible health issues of soy:

- Soy is a potent source of phytoestrogens that mimic estrogen and can lead to infertility and may promote breast cancer in adult women
- Drinking two glasses of soy milk daily for as little as one month can alter a woman's menstrual cycle
- Soy is high in goitrogens, substances that can block the normal functioning of the thyroid gland
- The processing of soy produces cancer-causing nitrosamines
- Soy foods contain high levels of aluminum, which is toxic to the nervous system

Note: *Infants must not be given soy milk (infant formula) as this can harm their sexual and reproductive development.*

Weight loss claims: Soy proponents claim that some studies show that people who regularly consume soy protein tend to weigh less and have less abdominal fat than those who don't. They claim that soy isoflavones (estrogen-like substances) reduce belly fat and protect against breast cancer, which is non-sense! Estrogenic compounds tend to increase belly fat and the presence of these isoflavones is one of the main reasons NOT to eat soy. As far as the breast cancer claim goes, a number of studies show that genistein (the main isoflavone) promotes the growth of breast cancer cells and tumours.

More Reading: If you want to read more about the dangers of soy, I suggest you read The Whole Soy Story by Kaayla T. Daniel – http://j.mp/1yng1o8

Coffee

The dangers or benefits of coffee are always good for a debate. Somehow, there seem to be two camps with opposing views. Coffee antagonists claim that it raises blood pressure (debatable), increases homocysteine levels (possibly true) and over-stimulates the adrenal glands. Coffee enthusiasts claim that it has many benefits, which include high levels of anti-oxidants, improved energy levels, cancer risk reduction, as well as protection from neurological diseases like Alzheimer's and Parkinson's disease.

If you like your coffee, I suggest that you stay with it, but do try to moderate your intake to no more than three or four cups a day. Also consider the following:

- Try to drink filtered instead of instant coffee because instant coffee contains chemicals and sometimes even gluten

- Avoid decaffeinated coffee if you can; the chemicals used to remove the caffeine from the coffee beans, which include Methylene Chloride and Ethyl Acetate, are definitely not health additives

Daily-use items to avoid

Commercial table salt

Normal table salt comes with some additives that make it not completely natural. Remember that natural salt is not white! Most salt of this kind has an anti-caking agent added to prevent the salt from clumping. These anti-caking agents can be:

- Calcium silicate
- Sodium alum inosilicate (contains aluminum)

- Magnesium carbonate (not regarded as toxic to eat, but burns the skin and eyes and causes gastric irritation if swallowed)

In addition, when salt is iodised it usually has a potassium salt such as potassium iodide or sodium iodide added, along with some dextrose, to prevent the potassium iodide from oxidising.

There is too much legislative laxity around anti-caking agents for anyone trying to heal their gut to take a chance with them. Therefore, I recommend that you make use of pure sea salt or Himalayan salt crystals. The extra cost is well worth it.

Toothpaste

Normal off-the-shelf toothpaste is not the best stuff to put in your mouth or gut. It contains a number of chemicals that can damage your gut. It should be obvious; never swallow toothpaste. In fact, washing your mouth out with water after brushing is probably a good idea. Consider switching to a natural toothpaste.

Here are some of the chemicals that may be in your toothpaste:

- Sodium fluoride, a poison that damages your gut and can cause nausea, vomiting or diarrhea. A Harvard University study found that it lowers children's IQ. Not the kind of stuff a sensible person would want near their body. This does not seem to worry the U.S. authorities. In 2012, so much fluoride was added to the U.S. water supply that a staggering 67% of people in America drank water with added sodium fluoride or fluorosilicic acid.

- Dyes for colouring, which are often made from petroleum products.

- Foaming agents that make bubbles as you brush can be deadly. The most common chemical for making bubbles is SLS (sodium laurel sulfate) and its derivatives. These potent chemicals have been linked to a number of reports that indicate increased cancer risks.

- Triclosan, a pesticide and antibacterial agent that has been linked to many health and environmental safety issues.

- Silica, used as an abrasive to clean tooth enamel. It is also combined with cellulose in 'tooth whitening' products.

Mouthwash

Most commercial mouthwashes contain similar chemicals to the ones listed above. Use with caution and never swallow mouth-wash.

Safety rules for brushing teeth or using mouthwash:

- Consider using an organic or natural product
- Use as little as possible to get the job done
- Never swallow the stuff
- Spit it out properly, then rinse your mouth out with plenty of water and spit that out too

Tinned foods

Be careful of food sold in tins as tinned food is devoid of any live components. The tins are also lined with a protective plastic that further increases health risks. The plastic protective lining used in most tinned food contains Bisphenol A (BPA) as well as other plastic pollutants. BPA has become a major health problem because it mimics natural hormones such as estrogen and disrupts hormone balance.

Plastic bottles and containers

These are bad for you! There is a huge commercial enterprise aimed at making and selling all manner of plastic utensils that are so convenient for us.

Plastic water bottles are a good example. You can use them over and over again, no problem. No! Plastic is made from chemicals that are not good for you, one of which is BPA. Don't pack or leave food in plastic wrap unless you want the chemicals in the wrap to be part of your next meal.

Don't:
- Heat food in plastic containers as it greatly increases the levels of plasticisers in the food
- Put warm food into a plastic container
- Use and especially re-use cheap plastic items. As a rule, the cheaper or flimsier the plastic the more dangerous it is to your health.

Whenever possible, store your food in glass containers.

Antacids

Many of these over-the-counter, so-called heartburn remedies contain aluminum, which can cause constipation.

Over-cooked foods

Avoid foods cooked at high temperatures, especially if cooked with vegetable oil (such as peanut, corn, and soy oil). Over-heating food like eggs oxidises cholesterol and turns it rancid.

CHAPTER 17

GUT HEALTH

One of the outcomes of eating real food and increasing your insulin sensitivity is improved gut health. Many people live with a damaged gut, never suspecting that a 'leaky gut' is the spark that lights the fire of many illnesses, including the 80 or more auto-immune diseases.

Your gut is the largest point of contact between your body and the outside world. In fact, the inside of your gut is also outside your body. As unlikely as it sounds, your skin and gut are both totally exposed to the outside world. The big difference between your skin and your gut is the surface area they cover. Gut surface area is many times larger than your skin and covers about half the area of a badminton court.

In your gut, all that stands between you and the outside world is a single layer of cells. These cells, called epithelial cells, make up the gut mucosa, which guard the outside of your gut wall. The integrity of this barrier is crucial for your health and it often becomes damaged by the food that passes though it.

The health of your gut is important and a leaky gut can influence your health in many ways:

- Poor skin almost always reflects a damaged gut
- Painful joints are often caused by a leaky gut

- Mood swings can often be triggered by a leaky gut
- Low thyroid hormone levels could be caused by a leaky gut

Constipation

A simple test of gut health is regularity of bowel movements. Normal bowel movements should occur daily, without strain and without the need for anti-constipation medication. Stools should conform to a normal shape and consistency.

- Chronic constipation is a warning about poor gut health
- Daily, easy, chemically unaided bowel motions are a necessity
- Your gut health affects your mood and mental state
- Psyllium husks are an ideal gut health promoter and bowel motion regulator

Stool science

- Stool shape and size is an important indicator of your gut health (you can follow this link to see the Bristol Stool Chart for examples: http://j.mp/1QHRGM6)
- Normal stools are soft and sausage-shaped
- Pellet or stony stools are a sign of constipation
- Consistently black stools are an important health warning and need medical investigation

Your second brain: Your gut is so important it even has a 'brain' of its own, making the gut the only organ in the body that has its own nervous system. Some scientists call it the 'second brain' because it can sometimes change your mind without you even realising it.

While the nerve cells in your head are concentrated in an organ called a brain, the nerves of the gut are widely distributed along its length. There are still a lot of them, though; an estimated 200 to 500 million nerve cells, which is a lot more than that of a mouse (71 million) and at least the size of the brain of a rat (200 million).

This nervous system has a direct connection to the brain, called the vagus nerve, along which it sends and receives messages. The nervous system of the gut responds to emotions and experiences. We have all experienced this gut-brain connection at times of great stress or as 'butterflies' when we are nervous. Surprisingly, tests have shown that the gut sends far more information to the brain than the other way around. Poor health can send signals to the brain that result in depression, yet another reason for you to care about your gut health.

This means that the gut somehow dictates to the brain. Despite this deluge of information being transmitted from gut to brain, little of the information is perceived consciously. Conscious or not, these messages have real effects, for example stimulation of the vagus nerve in depressives, who have been resistant to any other therapy, makes them feel better. With all this connectivity to the brain as well as its extensive body defense requirements, it is almost unthinkable that the gut is not playing a critical role in mind states, says Emeran Mayer, director of the Center for Neurobiology of Stress at the University of California, Los Angeles.

Serotonin: The gut concentrates about 90% of the body's 'feel good' neurotransmitter serotonin. We know that serotonin is directly involved in mood balance and that we can make someone happier by raising serotonin levels. It is very much part of the successful functioning of popular mood-lifting drugs like Zoloft and a host of others.

Bacteria communicate with your brain: It is becoming increasingly clear that the bacteria in our gut can affect our thinking in ways that were never considered before. Have you ever had one of those urgent, anxious sugar cravings? The kind where all self-restraint goes out the window and you end up scoffing mounds of sugar-laden foods, only to be drowned by waves of remorse a short while later? Would you believe that scientists are busy proving that some sugar cravings are initiated by gut bacteria? They think that hungry, sugar-loving bacteria produce neuroactive chemicals that initiate signals from the enteric nervous system to the brain. These announce in no uncertain terms that you NEED SUGAR!

Gut health: In addition to consuming some probiotics, either in the form of fermented foods or as supplements, and avoiding the consumption of gut irritants, adding a regular dose of psyllium husks to your diet can make a real difference to the health of your gut. Taken once a day in a glass of water, a heaped tablespoon of psyllium husks will ease constipation, soften stools and promote the growth of gut-healthy bacteria. While I admit that initially the mixture is a little repulsive in look and feel, it has almost no taste and once you get used to it, becomes quite manageable.

Biotics: Pre, Pro and Post

The various types of pre- and probiotics are intended to correct imbalances in the types and quantities of bacterial colonies that grow in our gut. Postbiotics are produced by bacteria and have value to the bacteria themselves, as well as to the body that hosts them.

Our modern, sugar-laden diet promotes the growth of un-friendly and unhealthy bacteria in the gut. Imagine this kind of imbalance as a garden that is not well tended and consequently becomes weed infested. Removing weeds and re-growing good vegetation requires the right fertilisers, time and consistent effort.

Successfully balancing and rejuvenating your gut bacteria will, in the same way as the garden, require time and consistency.

Prebiotics

Prebiotics are indigestible substances that aid or support the growth of the beneficial bacteria inside or on our bodies. The prebiotics available today almost exclusively target the organisms living inside our gut. However, recent developments point to a new area of skin prebiotics with creams containing prebiotics specifically designed to nourish beneficial skin bacteria.

Most prebiotics are made from fibre that our systems cannot digest. The beneficial bacteria in our gut ferment these fibres to provide them with nourishment to help them grow. The bacteria that digest prebiotics are found in the colon (large intestine). Food normally passes through the small intestine quickly to allow time for this kind of fermentation in the large intestine.

In general, prebiotics will aid the growth of bifido bacteria and lactobacilli, two groups of beneficial bacteria that enhance food digestion and boost immune functions.

The two major types of prebiotics are short-chain and long-chain. Short-chain prebiotics, the best known of which is FOS (fructo-oligosaccharide), are fermented quickly because of their small molecular size. Because they ferment more quickly, short-chain prebiotics work mostly in the ascending colon. Long-chain prebiotics, like inulin and resistant starch, provide nourishment to the bacteria in the transverse and descending colons.

Resistant starch: This is a special type of carbohydrate that cannot be broken down into sugars during digestion. Resistant starch is found in foods like potatoes, pasta, beans and lentils. A good way to take resistant starch is in the form of potato starch, which you can mix with water. Bacteria in the large intestine can break resistant starch down into short-chain fatty acids such as butyrate.

Butyrate: One of the beneficial effects of eating prebiotic fibres is that they increase the concentration of butyric acid (butyrate) in the colon. This short-chain fatty acid has been studied in mice, where it has been shown to increase heat production (metabolism) and to reduce cholesterol and triglyceride levels. The mice were rendered insulin-resistant before the trial and started the trial obese. A high butyrate diet increased their insulin sensitivity and reduced their body weight.

Note: Besides taking your prebiotic fibre every day, butter is the best dietary source of butyrate, which got its name from butter.

Probiotics

These are designed to deliver live beneficial bacteria to the gut. I suggest that you consider making yourself fermented foods that deliver living probiotics in much higher doses. Home-made fermented foods are a staple of just about every known culture and besides tasting a whole lot better than a store-bought pill, they also cost a lot less.

If you want to buy your probiotics, you will find a profusion of different kinds available on the market. I suggest you try some different brands over a period, hopefully while you develop the skills required to make your own fermented food.

One of the reasons there are so many different kinds of commercial probiotics is that packaging a probiotic formulation that actually delivers live bacteria after being shipped and then standing on a store shelf at various temperatures, represents quite a challenge.

Besides the logistical challenges, any live bacteria that actually make it into the mouth of a consumer still have to survive the passage through the acid bath in the stomach.

Here are some of the probiotic bacteria you should find in good supplements:

Lactobacilli, listed below, have proven scientific value. Some of them may also be effective against bladder infections.

- Acidophilus
- Reuteri
- Rhamnosus
- Casei
- Fermentum

Bifidobacteria make up about 25% of bacteria found in the colons of adults. The animalis variety is found in high levels in fermented dairy products and has been shown to survive gastric transit.

- Bifidum
- Longum
- Animalis

Postbiotics

These kinds of substances are produced by the bacteria themselves and are not normally taken orally. There have been some attempts to create oral postbiotics using heat-killed bacteria.

This method delivers the beneficial substances, which include butyrate, without the possible danger of administering live bacteria.

Practically speaking, at the moment you cannot take a post-biotic but you can ensure the promotion of their growth in your gut by taking pre- and probiotics and ensuring that you stay away from sugar and junk food.

The other stuff missing from Banting

You could stop reading this book at the end of this chapter, but there are still two crucial areas of your health that need attention. Two areas that, for a small investment in time and attention, will give you a massive return on your investment. These are areas that Banting misses completely and they are Mind and Movement.

CHAPTER 18

WHAT BANTING FORGOT: MIND AND MOVEMENT

Banting is a concept that deals with the stuff that goes into your mouth; it is blind to two other areas that are profoundly connected to your health and your enjoyment of life.

One way to visualise this deficit is as a wheel composed of three equal parts that need to work together in order for it to turn effortlessly. A fully enjoyable life results when there is a balance between sustenance (Meal), brain health (Mind) and activity (Move). Many of us live an unbalanced life, often unaware that these areas are out of balance.

Here is a simple equation that represents a life-goal that everyone should work toward: living a long and healthy life.

Healthspan = lifespan

While this simple equation should be everyone's goal, many of us reach old age physically diminished, propped up by the pills and potions of modern medicine. There is a pervasive belief that it's normal for humans to degrade physically as they age. The accepted norm holds that we are designed to wear out, become unstable, infirm and weak in our old age; in reality, with proper maintenance, most humans can live longer and stay stronger well into their old age.

In ancestral times, staying with the tribe as it moved was a matter of life or death; young ones could be carried, but older members who could not keep up would be left behind to perish. It was not in the tribe's best interests to lose its elders because access to their patience and experience would confer a significant survival advantage to the tribe. This means that the preservation of vitality into old age acted as an important evolutionary driver.

If this line of thinking is correct, we should still carry this ability. Interestingly, some statistics from the New York City Marathon clearly back this up. Beginners who start running at the age of 18 run faster each year until they peak at about the age of 30; from then onward, they begin to slow down, usually by a few seconds a year.

Since the runners become slower each year, can you guess when they actually reach the point that they run slower than in their teenage years? For example, does it seem likely that a 50-year-old would be able to outrun herself as a teenager?

You bet she would.

The amazing thing is that, on average, runners continue to run faster than their teenage selves until about the age of 65! This clearly shows that with the correct maintenance, our bodies are designed to keep moving at the same speed as younger tribe members until well into old age. However, take a look at some of the 60-year-olds you know and you will quickly realise that many of them are not up to a brisk walk round the block, let alone fit enough to run a marathon.

Modern life

The way we live our modern life – our poor nutrition, stress and lack of activity – leads us to an old age full of weakness and incapability. Machines transport us everywhere; the longest walk we take is either to or from the car park or a trip down the passage to the toilet. We take pills for everything. A study of American adults over the age of 65 showed that 90% used at least one medication and 40% used five or more. In contrast to the inactivity of our bodies, our minds are ceaselessly exercised by a torrent of visual, auditory and mental distractions that ensure we need a handful of pills every day to make it to old age.

It doesn't have to be this way.

Meal, mind, move

The small effort of balancing these 3Ms will go a long way to making your life more enjoyable and meaningful. It will greatly increase your chances of a longer, healthier life.

In the coming chapters, I outline in some detail the steps you can take to heal your **mind** and **move** your body every day in an unstressful, non-obsessive but meaningful way.

CHAPTER 19

MIND MANAGEMENT: STRESS AND SLEEP

'Our life is the creation of our mind.'

Buddha

There is more to health than just looking good; good health is about balance i.e., the balance between mind and body, a deceptively simple concept that so many of us seem to get wrong. Most commonly, we obsess about a certain aspect of the whole and as a result unbalance ourselves. The mind is central to who we are and our sense of wellbeing. The Banting way of life all but ignores this aspect of health which, to me, is too vital to leave to chance.

Missing persons

A few years ago there was an older guy in my gym whom I admired from a distance. Tall and rangy, good-looking enough to be a model, with the craggy visage that is *de rigueur* for the men we expect to see in aspirational advertisements about investments or luxury cars. His long grey-flecked locks, too long for the boardroom, reached his muscled back and chiseled shoulders. He would glide the tiled floors of the change rooms, buck-naked, absolutely at peace with his lithe body and swinging penis. Yet despite all this physical glory, he would never smile.

Then suddenly, he was gone.

I asked around for a few weeks but no one knew what had happened to him. I forgot about him until one day, months later, someone was telling me about his cousin, a fit guy who had died suddenly. This cousin was a bulimic who kept his weight under control by self-induced vomiting. He was always in and out of dentists' rooms because his teeth had eroded from stomach acid and he never smiled. That's how I realised he was talking about 'my guy' from the gym, so beautiful on the outside yet so sick in other ways.

Looking after your mind

Protecting and nurturing your brain should be your number one priority and there are two main areas that need attention:

- Stress
- Sleep

Reducing your stress levels and increasing your sleep time will make a profound difference to your health and outlook on life.

The effects of stress

Walking around with a clenched jaw, racing thoughts, rapid shallow breathing and a sense of urgency are not fun for any-one, yet it happens to all of us at some time or another. Unfor-tunately, the nervous system we have inherited from our primate ancestors is not well adapted to the stress of modern life. The chronic or unremitting stress most of us live with has many negative long-term effects, which include:

- A weakened immune system
- Damage to the brain and nervous system

- Faster aging
- Leaky gut
- Heart damage
- Overweight
- Reduced ability of the gut to absorb nutrients and minerals and the knock-on effects of these deficiencies

Chronic stress

My sister (bless her) uses the word chronic to mean 'bad'; in her mind, chronic stress means a lot of stress. However, in medical terms chronic simply means 'ongoing and not getting better'.

Chronic stress is woven into the background noise of our daily lives and is a major health threat, especially because our bodies are not designed to deal with it. Instead, we are wired to react to sudden life or death events, the kinds of challenges that are resolved in seconds or minutes. For example, being chased by a lion is immediately stressful. This kind of stress is resolved quickly: the lion wins or, if not, the threat goes away quickly and stress levels drop.

The opposite occurs in modern life. Most of our stressors are ever-present such as work, traffic, queues, financial worries, family pressures, and so on. These chronic stresses cause our engines to be fuelled by something they were never designed to run on.

Cortisol – the stress hormone

Cortisol, an adrenal hormone, is the fuel of stress. Despite being involved in many functions in the body, such as maintaining blood pressure levels and regulation of the immune system, cortisol and adrenaline are also key players in the body's reaction to stress. As a result, cortisol is known as the 'stress hormone'. Chronic stress can be measured in the blood and shows up as high cortisol and low DHEA (Dehydroepiandrosterone) levels.

When cortisol is squirted into the blood during an immediately stressful situation, it acts to slow digestion and reduce gut absorption. Blood is diverted from the gut to the muscles where it can do more immediate good. This action seems sensible when the aim is to stay alive. The gut can digest the food later. However, when cortisol levels in the blood remain chronically high, the gut becomes leaky, worsening any auto-immune disease you may have.

You can get your doctor to measure your cortisol levels, often done with a simple spit test. Blood cortisol levels usually mirror stress levels which can be monitored periodically to measure how well your stress management is working.

Stress affects your entire body

Many internal body processes are 'automatic' and proceed without our knowledge or control. Our nervous system is an example. It is made up of two opposing systems – 'fight or flight' and 'feed and breed' – that normally work in equilibrium, but in stressful conditions control shifts to the 'speed me up' fight or flight system. This results in the typical 'stressed out' state we so often exist in. These two systems are called the sympathetic and parasympathetic nervous systems, respectively. The stress reduction strategies outlined in this section strive to reduce the influence of your unconscious 'fight or flight' dominance in favour of the more restful 'feed and breed' system.

Stress affects your gut

Stress also affects your gut. Think of that queasy feeling you have before the big exam or the loss of appetite, and maybe even explosive diarrhea, before the big interview. Some of us lose our appetite in stressful situations, others can't stop eating. Either way, it's the gut telling the brain how to act.

Simply thinking of a stressful incident or replaying a social slight can affect your body. As the negative thought goes through your mind, your blood pressure rises, blood is diverted away from your gut and digestion slows down.

A recent study looked at how common stress, such as multi-tasking, affects the gut. The test subjects spoke on the phone and, at the same time, tried to listen to someone standing next to them asking them a question. This is a situation we can all relate to. The researchers then measured the change in mineral absorption in each test subject's gut. What they found was astounding. The stress of trying to multi-task halved gut absorption in the test subjects.

What's more, the absorption deficit persisted for more than two hours, even after the stress was withdrawn. It does not take much imagination to apply this one simple stress and its effects on your gut on a typical Monday morning.

Stress also affects the bugs living in our gut. They feel our stress and a stressful event can decimate gut bacterial populations, similar to what happens on a larger scale to soldiers in combat. A Russian study of pilots in dangerous combat missions found that the stress of combat could totally wipe out all the bugs in a pilot's gut.

Adrenal stress

Cortisol, the stress hormone, is produced by your adrenal glands. Normally your adrenals will raise cortisol levels during a sudden emergency. This response is aimed at boosting your energy levels so that you can escape the emergency. However, the stress of modern life causes an over-production of cortisol. As a result, some people live their lives with elevated levels of cortisol, which is really bad for their health.

It is said that 'the adrenals listen to what your heart tells your brain'. This means that a lower, steadier heart rate drops your cortisol levels and thus reduces your stress. Many of the stress-management methods I suggest also do exactly that.

Stress makes you old

Stress makes you age faster. It has been shown that there is a strong relationship between perceived stress and the rate at which you age. Nobel prize-winning biologist, Elizabeth Blackburn, measured stress at a cellular level using mothers caring for their children in ICU. Her data indicated that they aged about 10 years faster than women who did not have to deal with this kind of stress.

Managing your relationship with stress

Fact: You cannot avoid stress. So often we hear well-meaning stress management advice that cautions us to 'avoid stress'. Unfortunately, this is impossible for most of us to do. Stress is part of modern life and can only be avoided by impractical means, such as retreating to a cave in the wilderness.

Root out the little stresses of daily life

The first step you can take is to identify things that stress you in daily life and, where possible, make adjustments to reduce them. Write down your stressors, identify the ones that you have control over and fix them as best you can.

For example, if you find the traffic on the way to work stressful, make an arrangement to avoid it. If missing deadlines is stressful, find a way to do your work on time. Just the act of recognising the small things that cause you stress is a step in the right direction.

Ways to de-stress

Here are some great ways to de-stress. Try them out and see which ones work best for you. My list is not exhaustive; please add your own methods if you need to. I have, however, specified some non-negotiable de-stress techniques, which I call the 'Must dos'. You have to try to make these a part of your lifestyle in the future.

There is also a section of other suggested options that you can review and select from.

Must do

- Control your breathing
- Eat mindfully
- Control your self-talk

Strongly suggested

- Get back to nature
- Nurture your friendships and relationships
- Get hugged every day

- Meditate
- Go on a low-info diet
- Eat dark chocolate
- Sweat

Controlled breathing

Slow or controlled breathing is an effective way to reduce stress. Regular slow breaths signal to your brain that all is well and, if done properly, will induce a relaxation response. In this way, you can convert the rapid, shallow breathing of someone under stress to that of a relaxed person.

Controlled breathing is often the result of many stress-relieving activities like meditation, prayer, reading a book or listening to music. Once you learn a controlled breathing technique, you can use it when you experience high stress to tell your brain that you are okay. You can use it as often as you like; it will work for you in the traffic, in bed or in the office.

The relaxation response

This term, coined by Harvard physician Dr Herbert Benson in the 1970s, was based on his work which suggested that we have a natural response designed to relax us, just as we have the fight or flight response. He believed that a mental device such as a sound, a prayer, staring at a scene and adopting a passive attitude that put stressful thoughts aside, would produce relaxation irrespective of the circumstances. This meant that it could be used anywhere, not just in quiet situations. Today even mainstream medicine agrees and has found similar benefits. An example is Breath Focus, presented in a 2015 article published by the Harvard Medical School, which describes a breath control method to lower stress levels.

Control your breath to:

- Reduce stress
- Lower anxiety levels
- Drop blood pressure
- Lower heart rate

Making time for breath control

Breath control is a vital tool in your stress management toolbox. Have you ever seen Captain America in action? He uses his brightly-painted shield to deflect sharp objects intended to harm him. Breath control is your shield.

Use your shield as you feel your stress begin to rise. Do it, too, at other times convenient for you, for example: in your car in the traffic; before you start work or a meeting; and in bed. Another really important time is just before meals; it only takes a few seconds and will improve digestion and your enjoyment of the meal.

Signs that you are winning

Controlled breathing stimulates the 'rest and relax' part of your nervous system. When you do it properly, you may feel some physical sensations such as a running nose, rosy face or a sense of body warmth. If you often feel cold, breathing like this will help to warm you up.

Buteyko breathing

I want to teach you a 'lite' version of Buteyko breathing. Ukrainian physiologist Konstantin Buteyko developed it as an asthma treatment, but it also has great value in other areas.

Buteyko believed that a modern lifestyle and open-mouth breathing lead to higher carbon dioxide levels in the blood. Higher carbon dioxide levels constrict blood vessels and reduce oxygen levels in places like the hands and feet. When you breathe the Buteyko way, you warm up, think more clearly, have higher energy levels and better sleep patterns.

Nose breathing is the key because it lowers carbon dioxide levels and raises nitrous oxide levels, which open the lung passages and improve blood flow. It will almost always unblock blocked noses.

You are in no danger of running out of oxygen

Buteyko breathing will not affect your oxygen levels!

Your urge to breathe is driven by levels of carbon dioxide in your blood. If these are too high, they will unnecessarily reduce the pauses between your breaths, making you over-breathe. Over time, breathing the Buteyko way will give you better body oxygenation and lower stress levels.

Test your carbon dioxide levels

Here is a simple way for you to find out if your carbon dioxide levels are too high. It can be done anywhere and at almost any time. All you need is a timer with a second hand.

Here's how to do it:

- Sit comfortably on a chair
- Breathe out normally
- Use thumb and finger to pinch your nose closed
- Start timing
- Hold your breath
- Wait until you feel the first definite desire to take a breath
- Read the timer
- Let go of your nose and breathe in

It is not a 'hold your breath' contest! What you are measuring is the time it takes before you consciously feel the need to take a breath. If you were in a breath-holding competition, you could hold your breath for much longer.

A control pause of 20 seconds or less points to a high carbon dioxide level; over 25 is fair; and over 30 seconds is a good result.

It is not a sign of fitness. In fact, most fit people have poor control pauses because they over-breathe when they train. I tested some elite cyclists a while ago and once they stopped trying to win the breath-holding contest, most of them came in at 15 seconds or below. As fit as they were, their breathing was driven by carbon dioxide and once they trained using Buteyko methods, most of them had improved race performances.

Work on your control pause

I work on my control pause all day! So should you.

Do this often: whenever you have a moment during the day, consciously don't breathe in and when you feel the urge to take a breath, wait an extra few seconds before you do. Over time, the gap between your breaths will increase and so will your control pause.

Buteyko breathe all the time

Here's how to do controlled breathing the Buteyko way.

First, I suggest that you breathe through your nose all the time or at least as often as you can manage. Second, do the exercise below when you need to de-stress or are about to eat a meal, go to bed, etc.

Points to remember:

- You can do this anywhere
- Always breathe through your nose
- Never take full chest stretching breaths in
- Never force all the air out of your lungs
- You don't have to hold your nose if you don't want to

Buteyko controlled breathing exercise

- Get as comfortable as you can
- Close your mouth
- Take a normal, relaxed breath in and out through your nose (don't breathe deeply)
- Now hold your breath or block your nose and do a slow mental countdown from five to one
- Then unblock your nose and take a gentle breath in and out
- Hold your breath again or block your nose for a slow count of five (NB: It is important to breathe comfortably, so if you find this pause difficult, you can reduce or omit the pause)
- Repeat this process for between two to four minutes

- If you become short of breath, keep breathing gently until you feel comfortable again

There are many online resources that will provide you with more detail about this method.

Here's a link to get you started: http://j.mp/1Fhma2g

Nadi shodhana (Nadi shodan)

Nadi shodhana is from *pranayama*, Sanskrit for the 'extension of life energy through breath'. We will learn a version of pranayama that uses the nose (nadi) purification (shodhana). It has a similar action to the Buteyko method discussed above.

Also known as Alternate Nostril Breathing, nadi shodhana is a form of breathing that has been shown to produce relaxation and reduce heart rate. It has also been found to have beneficial effects on heart rate variability as well as on improving problem-solving abilities.

In this method, you rhythmically alternate breathing between the left and right nostrils, with pauses between both in and out breaths. There are many YouTube videos showing the technique; browse through them and find a method that you're comfortable with. This link will take you to YouTube and start your search: http://j.mp/1FhmqOF

The basic method is as follows:

- Sit comfortably with your spine erect and shoulders relaxed
- Place your left hand on your left knee, palms open, thumb and index finger gently touching at the tips
- Place the tip of the index finger and middle finger of the right hand in between the eyebrow

- Place the ring finger and little finger on the left nostril, and the thumb on the right nostril
- Press your thumb down on the right nostril and breathe out gently through the left nostril
- Breathe in from the left nostril and then press the left nostril gently with the ring finger and little finger
- Removing the right thumb from the right nostril, breathe out from the right
- Breathe in from the right nostril and exhale from the left
- You have now completed one round of nadi shodhana pranayama
- Continue inhaling and exhaling from alternate nostrils

SUGGESTED: Mindful eating

Don't eat on the move!

Never grab a quick bite and don't eat when you're stressed. Rushed eating sends a message to your gut telling it that you are under stress.

As you've just learned, stress affects two major areas of digestion: it lowers the ability of your gut to absorb nutrients from the food you eat; it also negatively affects the good bacteria in your gut, sometimes even killing them off.

During a video lecture, Marc David, a specialist in the psychology of eating, recounts the story of one of his patients, Dr X. Dr X believed that he ate well but nevertheless experienced intense indigestion after every meal. Despite having access to many medical specialists, he had lived with abdominal discomfort for almost 20 years. Dr X's daily fare was McDonald's for breakfast and lunch, eaten in his car in the McDonald's parking lot, in order to save time. For dinner, he would consume a take-out in front of the TV.

He insisted that he was happy with his lifestyle and would not consider changing it. Amazingly, Marc David did not try to persuade Dr X to eat healthy food (as I would have done). What he prescribed was a simple eating slow-down. All he asked Dr X to do was to spend more time over each of his junk food meals and to slow down with some deep breaths before starting to eat.

Two weeks later Dr X called Marc to say that his digestive issues were completely cured. On top of this, once he had slowed his eating down, he found that he could actually taste the Big Macs, which now tasted terrible to him, and he switched to healthier food as a result.

Slow down when you eat

Eating under duress, be it anxiety, time pressures or any other stressor, is bad for your gut. Tests performed to study stressful eating have shown that stress can reduce absorption by as much as 50% for up to two hours afterward.

You are stress eating when you eat:

- On the run
- Standing up
- In the car
- Quickly
- On autopilot

Eating mindfully

The concept of mindful eating comes from Buddhist teachings about how to eat. Before eating, Buddhists consider the food they are about to eat and where it comes from. They also chew their food carefully, savouring the tastes and textures.

Marc David suggests a pause to regulate breathing before starting to eat. You could use the Buteyko technique mentioned in the Controlled breathing section, or just simply, mindfully slow your breathing. Try to be present in the act of eating. Don't eat on autopilot, not even tasting the food that you swallow.

How to eat mindfully

1. Control your breathing
2. Consider the food on your plate; try to be grateful for the food that you are about to eat
3. Be present in the act of eating
4. Chew each mouthful properly
5. Feel the texture of your food, explore the taste of it
6. Make a conscious effort to slow down

Control your self-talk

*'Don't let the noise of others' opinions
drown out your inner voice'*
Steve Jobs

Ever done any self-attacking?

You know, those times when you think mean thoughts about yourself or insult and undermine yourself. I suppose we are all guilty of doing this from time to time, but if it's the norm, then this kind of behaviour is bad for your stress levels.

Self-attacking ties in with self-esteem. Self-esteem is about how you see yourself, your skills, abilities and overall value. Your level of self-esteem not only guides your behaviour, it has also been shown to predict health and wellbeing.

If you have a poor opinion of yourself, or if you have a tendency to berate and insult yourself, then you have to work on this area in order to manage and reduce your stress levels. Additionally, this kind of behaviour reduces your ability to handle other stressful situations that you may have to deal with as part of daily life.

Frame your self-attacker as someone else

Next time you have a self-attacking thought, stop and ask yourself: What if someone else had said that to you? Would you think differently about it then?

Then think about this: How would you feel if someone was following you around all day berating you with negative personal comments? Would you tolerate having this sort of person around you? Surely you would soon grow tired of the haranguing and negativity and try your best to avoid their bad company?

There is no reason to tolerate this type of behaviour, especially if you are inflicting it on yourself!

Restricting self-criticism

Do you think that you are hard on yourself? Do you tend to colour events and issues in a negative light?

Read these words:

- Useless
- Pathetic
- Stupid

- Worthless
- Ugly
- Inadequate

Does thinking about any of these words make you feel bad?

Well, you shouldn't feel that way. Self-criticism is not a good thing. Trust yourself and always choose praise over criticism. I ask the question again: Are you too hard on yourself?

> *'Too many people undervalue what they are,*
> *and overvalue what they're not.'*
> Internet postcard

Dr Melanie Fennell is a recognised expert on low self-esteem and she suggests that the best way to handle self-critical thoughts is with a three-step process:

Recognise, question, reframe

1: Recognise the negative

Catch the thoughts as they happen. Although you may find recognition to be difficult at first, be alert because self-critical thoughts can be triggered by certain situations or mental images. Learn to take notice of when you start feeling down about yourself. If you find this difficult, Fennel suggests setting a timer to go off at one-hour intervals and use this as the cue to ask yourself if you have had any self-critical thoughts over the past 60 minutes.

2: Question each negative thought

Ask yourself *why* you are thinking negative thoughts and try to seek a balanced alternative. You can try to do this as a trial lawyer questioning a witness would do by asking yourself:

- Are you certain of your facts?
- Are you jumping to conclusions?
- Are you being too hard on yourself and too easy on others?
- Are you taking the blame for things that were not your fault?
- Are you thinking in black and white and allowing yourself no leeway?

3: Reframe

Review your negative thoughts in a positive way. Then act according to the new way you are looking at them. Always treat yourself with respect.

Example: 'I'm useless, I only came fifth overall.'
Reframed: 'Nice job! I came in fifth and I just started playing.'

Of course, it is important not to lose touch with reality but putting a positive spin on things helps. Yes, you need to face your failures, but cast them as learning experiences or as some bad luck that was unfortunately directed at you.

Recognise biased thinking

We naturally add weight to ideas and thoughts that are consistent with our beliefs, just as we diminish those that aren't. Don't you hate people who openly show bias or prejudice? People who start sentences with: 'I can't stand …'?

Now what if you are biased against yourself? What if, by default, you perceive thoughts about yourself, as well as events that happen to you, in a negative way? Why do such a bad thing to yourself? Recognising and removing this in-built bias will make a huge difference to your self-esteem.

Don't think in a self-limiting way

'I can't do that!' How often have you told yourself that?

Love the skin you're in

You've heard it before: 'If you don't love yourself, then who will?' There is no way to get a body transplant and the only way you are ever going to leave your body is when you die. So you need to accept, love and appreciate yourself.

Give yourself credit

If you do well at something, take a mental bow. Give yourself the credit – don't be so quick to give the credit to luck, to someone else, or even to the intervention of a deity. Give yourself a pat on the back.

Avoid the perfect

Nothing in life is perfect. Neither are you, so cut yourself some slack and don't always expect yourself to be perfect. Everybody has blemishes and bad days and so can you. Don't ever allow yourself to recognise criticism as failure.

Be confident

Did you know that you can train yourself to have more self-confidence? If you think that you lack confidence, consider taking a self-confidence course. There are many available online and some of them are even free.

Here are some pointers to consider:

- Remember your achievements and successes. Make a list and read it if you feel your confidence slipping.
- Make a list of your personal goals and tick off any that you achieve.
- Divide your goals into small steps and focus on one step at a time.
- Celebrate each success as you tick it off.
- Get your support network involved in your successes or your failures.
- Smile at yourself in the mirror.

Back to nature

> *'... being connected to nature and feeling happy are, in fact, connected.'*
> From a study of nature connectedness and happiness

When last were you outdoors?

Our roots as humans are deeply embedded in the outdoors. However, most of us spend almost no time outside even though contact with nature makes us happy in such an elemental way. Contact with nature is not optional. We need this kind of connectedness, which we can never reproduce by immersing ourselves in a life of materialism or machines.

What is nature?

Nature is more than the plants and trees we find outdoors. Animals and weather are also an important part of nature. As humans, we are hardwired to connect with other mammals. Think of your emotions when seeing baby animals, how you feel when looking into the eyes of a puppy or lion cub.

Nature is also weather. We control our living environments so tightly that it abstracts us from the real weather outdoors. Granted that the weather outdoors may be unpleasant: hot, humid, cold or wet. How do you feel when you think of a sunny day, a gloomy sky or walking in the rain? Maybe we need to experience the feeling of being too hot or too cold?

Exposure to nature

Spending time in natural surroundings restores some of our capacity to handle the emotional and psychological stresses in our daily lives. It works this way for adults and kids alike. A Swedish study found that children who spent time playing outdoors closer to nature had better development in the areas of learning and understanding (cognitive development) than kids who played in concrete jungles.

The ability to control our moods and to delay gratification is called self-regulation. Frances Ming Kuo, a Professor of Natural Resources and Environmental Sciences, says that our ability to self-regulate is enhanced by being outdoors. She believes this is an essential component of good health.

Practical steps to de-stress outdoors

I hope that having read the two paragraphs above, you fully appreciate how much your health needs you to spend some time outdoors! When you do get a chance to be outdoors, try to do it barefoot as this will magnify your connection.

My wife

My wife recently started on a mindfulness, back-to-nature journey that I initially poo-pooed. We are lucky to live in the suburbs in a house that has a garden and a small outdoor living area – an area that we have, in the past, spent very little time living in. She changed all that. First for herself, by spending time in the garden during the day and also at night-time. I joined her, initially just to be polite as I would normally work or watch TV indoors before bedtime. These days, I never wear shoes at home, whereas previously the only time I would walk barefoot was on my way to bed. I now put my cellphone away, seldom watch TV, and rather spend my time outside. We often just lie on the grass and look at the stars, an activity I would have considered crazy in the past. It has worked for me; I can't believe how much more relaxed I feel and how much more I am enjoying life at home.

Depending on your situation, getting to a park or a natural outdoor environment may not be so simple. If you live in a concrete environment, where the only green stuff around you is the vegetable aisle in the supermarket, then you need to be creative in finding ways to chill out in nature. Is there a park or a rooftop garden where you can retreat to? Make a plan. There has to be a way for you to get your bare feet in the grass or your skin in the sun a few times a week.

Find a safe place where you can sit outdoors, lie on the ground and read a book or stare into space. You don't always need company to do this; sometimes the solitude of being alone is a tonic.

Don't stress too much about the weather. If it's cold outside, dress warmly but still do it! If it's too hot, just relax and sweat a little, it's good for you.

Walk barefoot

'The research done to date supports the concept that grounding or earthing the human body may be an essential element in the health equation along with sunshine, clean air and water, nutritious food, and physical activity.'
Journal of Environmental and Public Health

Read that quote carefully. It was written by a group of scientific specialists whose skills include cell biology, cardiology and neurosurgery.

Our modern footwear insulates us from the earth. The Grounding Movement maintains that being in contact with the earth is a critical part of wellness. They believe that grounding (or earthing) by walking barefoot allows for the transfer of electrons from the earth's surface into our bodies, balancing us electrically. Ever since humans walked the planet, this was our natural state.

Obviously, this is not something that most mainstream medical practitioners accept, but since walking barefoot in nature is one of my prescriptions for stress management, what do you have to lose by trying it? Get out of your shoes whenever you get the chance.

Love your pet

If you don't have a pet, maybe you should consider getting one? Or if you do, spend time with your pet as it will do you both a power of good. Spending time with other people's pets will also work for you. Studies show that animals can reduce tension and improve mood. Research has found that owning a dog can lower blood pressure, reduce stress hormones, and boost levels of feel-good chemicals in the brain.

Nurture friendships and relationships

I am sure that you already know that good friendship and family relationships are important. When your relationships go well, they can be a great de-stressor. When things go wrong in your relationships, they can also be a source of great stress.

The science is clear: better relationships translate into lower stress levels. The problem is how to conduct and maintain better relationships. Like any other action in your de-stress mission, you are going to have to work at it. And like so many things in life, the more sustained the effort you make, the better your results will be.

Friendships take effort and time. They also require turning the other cheek occasionally. Family relationships are even harder but good family time is always good for you and your stress levels.

'External relationships are improved and maintained through your expression of acceptance, peace, compassion and respect for all individuals in your environment…'
From the book Managing Stress

Try to connect with others emotionally, spiritually and mentally. Don't isolate yourself at home or at work as the stress of this may lead to feelings of depression and isolation. Wherever possible, surround yourself with like-minded people who make you feel good.

Where possible, avoid negative energy in your life. You must know people who drain you and suck your positive energy? Avoid them. Don't be afraid to refuse invitations to events you would rather not attend. Be like the parent in the aircraft safety drill, first put the oxygen mask on your own face before looking after other passengers around you.

Think carefully about the suggestions below; they are certain to help you build better relationships and a committed support system that will be there for you whenever you need to de-stress.

Try to:

- Be respectful to everyone around you
- Be kind to others
- Give credit to others
- Be positive towards your family and friends
- Forgive, let go of meaningless offenses and slights
- Learn to receive from others by being less fearful, and more open and accepting
- Don't be afraid to ask for help

SUGGESTED: Get hugged daily

Hugging is good for you! It's a scientific fact that hugging is good medicine.

A good hug releases oxytocin. Patting a dog does too. Oxytocin is a stress reduction hormone that works its magic by dropping blood cortisol levels.

Boost your oxytocin every day

In addition to hugging, other ways to boost oxytocin include:

- Holding hands
- Having an orgasm
- Getting a massage
- Giving a backrub
- Doing breathing exercises and meditation
- Getting touched lightly
- Giving or receiving praise

Dr Love's eight hugs a day

Paul Zak, an American neuro-economist, is probably the most enthusiastic oxytocin fan on the planet. He is also known as Dr Love because of his advice to always hug people as a means of raising oxytocin levels. If you want to know more about Dr Love, watch his TED talk: Paul Zak: Trust, morality – and oxytocin. It has been watched over a million times: http://j.mp/1DXL62v

Dr Love suggests that to keep your oxytocin levels high and thus lower your stress, you should make sure that you are hugged eight times a day. I am not sure if you can achieve that but there is no harm in trying!

Meditate

For stressful daily situations, use the breathing control methods explained in the section before this one. Meditation (for beginners at least), requires a quiet place as well as the intention to relax and quieten the mind.

If you don't meditate yet, now is the time to start! It's a great way to lower your stress levels. Meditation has been shown by medical studies, as well as by countless personal experiences, to lower blood pressure, protect heart health, improve digestion (yes, that's the gut we're trying to heal) and boost immunity.

There are literally thousands of ways to meditate and myriad schools that teach it. If you are new to meditation, there are many teaching resources you can use. You can also find a local teacher or a group to join. There are also plenty of courses and apps online that you can download.

You can also combine meditation with controlled breathing, as discussed in the previous section.

I am going to outline a simple six-step method developed by Malaysian-born entrepreneur and philanthropist Vishen Lakhiani. He runs a website, Mind Valley Academy, which has many useful resources. One of these is his Six Phase Meditation Method, which he describes as a distillation of hundreds of books on personal growth. He calls it (rather modestly) 'The world's simplest, science-based meditation and mindfulness technique'. You can find more here: http://j.mp/1Nup2lX

The 6-phase meditation

There is a full video explanation by Vishen on YouTube, which you can find here: http://j.mp/1O1ESkU

Here, in brief, are the six steps:

Preparation: relaxation

Lack of tension and achieving comfort is your goal. Sit in a comfortable chair or lie flat with your head on a small pillow. Play some calming instrumental music at a low volume.

Then physically relax your body. Start by relaxing your scalp and, once it has relaxed, relax your eyelids, then flow gently down your body, relaxing each part as you go.

1) Connection

Focus on your consciousness; see it as a white light surrounding your body. Expand the light to encompass your suburb, then your town, then the world. Try to feel part of the whole.

2) Gratitude

Think of some of the things you should be grateful for, savour these things and feel the gratitude throughout your body.

3) Forgiveness

Think of someone who has done you wrong; try to imagine them in front of you. Apologise and ask for their forgiveness. Then forgive them.

4) Visualising success

Think of how you would like your life to turn out over the next few years. Feel how much better things will become in your life.

5) **Daily intention**

Visualise your day ahead; consider the things that you will enjoy during the day. See today as a wonderful gift.

6) **Blessing**

Summon your inner strength or the strength of a higher power. Ask for support, ask for luck and energy. Feel the support as your protective energy.

Now slowly bring yourself out of your meditation.

SUGGESTED: Go on a low-info diet

From the moment we awake until our eyes close at night we are bombarded with news and social updates. Does knowing this news help your life in any way? Does allowing yourself to be distracted by the whims of our sensationalist media or your friends and family serve you in any positive way?

Ask yourself this question: How much do you really need to know about foreign wars, terror attacks, lost planes, business indicators or the personal tragedies and triumphs of people you will never meet?

I strongly suggest that you consider going on an information diet as a stress management practice. It worked for me.

My low-info diet

From the beginning of the year, I stopped all news cold turkey. For the past few years, I permanently had a screen open on my laptop, streaming news from a 24-hour Internet news station. I would constantly flip between my work and the news feed, as if I was eager to read about some world-shattering event before the people around me could. Of course, I also had a news app on my smartphone and my car radio was permanently jammed on a 24-hour news station to ensure that I would miss nothing as I was driving.

Well, I stopped doing this and now I no longer float between the news website and my work. When I drive, classical music wafts from my car stereo and I make a conscious effort not to get angry in the traffic. I try to be courteous and, where possible, I make eye contact with other drivers and pedestrians. At home, the TV in my bedroom is unplugged and I eschew the addictive call of the news channels.

This makes me thoroughly under-informed. I rely on the people around me to tell me of world events and, most importantly, I don't waste time stressing about events that I have no control over.

The net effect of my information diet is that my stress levels are lower and I concentrate better on my work. I can now think almost as clearly as Rolf Dobelli, author of the best-selling book *The Art of Thinking Clearly* (Harper Collins).

Your low-info diet

Review your habits when it comes to the news and information. Think about how much time you spend reading news articles, blog posts and watching video news clips. Tune out from these as much as you can. Stop reading the newspapers.

While you're at it, think about your social media habits. If you are anything like so many of my patients, you probably spend too much time trawling Facebook and similar websites. Some people I know slavishly watch Twitter feeds, waiting for the opportunity to tweet something pithy and profound.

I am not suggesting that you delete your Facebook account! Rather, apply a sensible compromise that will work for you. Limit the time you spend on social media. Don't blindly go down rabbit holes dug by people who have too much time on their hands. Realise that you will run out of life long before the denizens of Facebook will run out of pointless, funny videos for you watch.

Suggestions:

- Work on your email in batches every few hours, resisting the urge to constantly check for new mail; also disable email notifications that distract and disturb you.
- Don't check your phone constantly – do it at regular intervals.
- Avoid news and social media updates that distract you from your work; rather set aside a time when you interact and respond to social media.

SUGGESTED: Eat dark chocolate

Besides the benefits to your heart from eating dark chocolate, there is also some scientific evidence that shows that dark chocolate is effective for lowering stress. Researchers have found that eating the equivalent of one average-sized dark choco- late bar each day for two weeks reduced levels of cortisol as well as the 'fight or flight' hormones in highly stressed people.

The findings add to a growing number of recently discovered potential health benefits of dark chocolate. For example, cocoa has been found to be rich in a class of antioxidants called flavo- noids, which have been linked to a number of health benefits.

Researchers are also investigating other compounds in dark chocolate that may offer other health benefits, such as improved insulin sensitivity, reduced blood pressure and improved mood.

Need to know

Before you rush off to buy some, there are a few important things that you need to know.

Avoid any dark chocolate that contains too much sugar. Many varieties of dark chocolate are similar to the popular brands of high-sugar milk chocolate. The dark chocolate you need to look for is normally clearly labeled with a cacao (cocoa) percentage. Go for the brands containing 80% or more of cacao. The higher the cacao percentage, the less sugar comes along for the ride and the more effective the chocolate will be at lowering stress.

My favourite dark chocolate is Lindt 85% which has high cocoa content and a meagre one gram of sugar in each square.

Unfortunately, the low sugar levels give this kind of chocolate a bitter taste. For eaters of 'normal' chocolate, this takes a bit of getting used to. Instead of starting with the 85% variety, rather work your way towards it by first eating 65% or 70% cacao for a few weeks. Initially these may also be a little bitter but stick with it for a few weeks before venturing into the higher percentages in order to acclimatise your taste buds.

Stress busting

A few studies have reported cortisol-lowering effects in test subjects. The initial study was done by researchers at the Nestle Research Center, which raised some eyebrows about impartiality. However, a subsequent study done in 2014 and reported in the *Journal of the American College of Cardiology* showed similar results. Researchers reported that eating some dark chocolate before a stressful event has an effect on the adrenal glands and reduces the levels of cortisol (the stress hormone) produced during the event.

I think that we can safely assume that dark chocolate has some de-stressing effect, which it exerts by reducing cortisol levels. I suggest that you indulge in a few squares of dark chocolate a few times a week, preferably after dinner when you are winding down.

Sweat!

> 'Sauna bathers most frequently cite stress reduction
> as the number one benefit of sauna use'
> Claim by various manufacturers of saunas

I thought long and hard about calling a regular sauna session a 'Must do' stress buster. But it is that important. A regular sweat is great for your stress levels.

We try our hardest to avoid sweating. It is just not done to sweat in polite company. People use anti-perspirants to block sweat glands and meet in rooms with air conditioners. From Hollywood's perspective, sweating is usually a sign of guilt. They often show scenes where the perpetrator pours sweat while the cops interrogating him are bone dry.

But you should sweat more when you can as it helps to excrete heavy metals from your body. In the right environment, sweating also reduces stress. I strongly recommend that you consider using the sauna and steam room as part of your de-stress programme. Use your time in the hot room to relax; it's a good time to use your meditation technique to further help relax your mind and body.

Some caution is required though; start slowly and increase your time in the hot room gradually. It is also prudent to have someone with you when you start in case you feel faint.

The bad press

When I was growing up, it seemed that steam rooms were somewhat sleazy places where old men and creeps sat and whispered under the cover of steam. Saunas had a better reputation but were less common. However, having spent quite some time visiting saunas and steam rooms over the past few years, I have had a complete reversal of opinion and now consider them to be some of the friendliest and most relaxing places in which to spend time. The people I meet, sitting semi-naked and pouring sweat, are almost invariably friendly. I often ask them why they do it and most of them say that it's the best part of their day.

Tom Cruise and the sauna

After the 911 catastrophe, many of the firefighters and emergency personnel who worked at Ground Zero were found to have high blood levels of heavy metals like arsenic, cadmium, lead and mercury. This was thought to be a result of their inhalation of toxin-laced smoke and dust from the burning materials in the buildings.

In 2003, actor Tom Cruise, as the co-founder of The New York Rescue Workers Detoxification Project, gave exposed workers access to a Scientology method for detoxification called the Purification Rundown. This has received both good and bad press but the main issue was that the saunas donated by Cruise worked. Some of the bad press was to do with the heavy niacin (vitamin B3) doses that were part of the Rundown programme. Niacin can result in some side-effects such as itchy skin or nausea.

However, some of the personnel on Cruise's programme had good results. A few of them even reported to have poured blue sweat when beginning the programme. This was identified as manganese, a heavy metal used in some of the structures of the World Trade Center.

Good press

Many studies exist in medical literature that underline the value of sweating as a form of detoxification. In a 2012 study, researchers identified 24 studies that looked at the detoxification effects of saunas. Using these as a base, they found that there was real value in sweating. The studies showed that high levels of heavy metals were excreted in the sweat of sauna users, sometimes even surpassing the levels in urine.

Give it a whirl

It does not matter if you start with the steam room or the sauna, give it a try. Besides the various public or private facilities, there are many home sauna systems available. Unlike the old days, when you needed to build a special room, there are new infrared-based units available that can be ordered online and self-installed. Infrared units plug into conventional power points and can even be purchased as single-user units that take up minimal space.

SLEEP

> *'...there will be sleeping enough in the grave....'*
> *Benjamin Franklin*

The words of Benjamin Franklin capture our modern attitude to sleep. We admire people who work hard and sleep little. This kind of behaviour often appears to be a core trait of many successful people.

Sleep is not wasted time

Unfortunately, we are wrong. Sleep is not wasted time. We cannot simply reduce our sleeping hours without cost to our health. We need our sleep, as does every living organism on earth, and our need for sleep remains the same as it has for millennia. Sleep cannot be deferred or 'caught-up' like an overdraft can be.

If you don't sleep, you will die. This happens literally in a condition known as fatal familial insomnia where increasing insomnia leads to death, usually in less than a year.

You need your sleep and, for many of us, sleeping properly is not easy. There are so many distractions and stresses that cause us to lose sleep. American adults, for example, get an average of 6.8 hours of sleep a night.

Do the math. Assuming that you miss an hour of sleep a night, over a year that translates to 15 days of missed sleep! That's vital body repair time you cannot afford to miss out on. You need to aim for eight hours of sleep a night to support your overall health.

Dangers of sleeping too little

Too little sleep also has negative health effects, some of which include:

- Immune system impairment
- Increase in inflammation
- Reduced performance of general tasks (on days following a poor night's sleep)
- Increased risk of heart disease
- Development of a pre-diabetic state
- Diabetes
- Premature aging
- Increased risk of dying from any cause

A lack of sleep also affects you mentally by making you over-emotional and causing you to think more slowly.

Make sleep a priority

Charles Czeisler, Professor of Sleep Medicine, says that while Benjamin Franklin may be right about deferring sleep until death, 'not sleeping will get you there a lot quicker'.

To maintain your health, you must adopt a mindset that prioritises sleep.

- Your goal is to sleep eight hours a day
- Stick to a regular bedtime on weekdays and weekends (kids have a specific bed-time and so should you)
- Develop a regular waking time on weekdays and weekends
- Maintain a firm stance when it comes to avoiding activities that interfere with your sleep times

Enabling sleep

Many of my patients complain, 'Doc, I just can't get to sleep.' And to be fair, we all have difficulty in getting to sleep at some time or another. There are ways for you to make it easier to sleep without resorting to the use of sleeping medications.

While your sleep can be disturbed for many reasons, some beyond your control, there are some factors that you do have control over. You need to make a concerted effort to manage these factors and construct the best possible sleep environment for yourself. Getting a dose of good sleep requires two ingredients:

· Good sleep foreplay
· A sleep-enhancing environment

Sleep foreplay

Why sleep foreplay? I like the word foreplay for the ritual before you actually go to sleep because it is a necessary and integral part of the main event, which is getting to sleep. Similar to other kinds of foreplay, failure to prepare properly can radically affect the quality of the main event. Try to view the time before you go to sleep as a period of preparation with certain regular steps.

Switching off your TV and your lights and then rolling over and expecting to fall asleep is asking too much of your mind and your body. How can you expect to transition from an alert, wakeful state to a sleeping state in a few minutes? You can't. Research shows that using an electronic device an hour before bed can delay sleep by over an hour.

Your sleep foreplay should start at least an hour before bedtime. It will prepare your mind and body for the coming sleep event. Have a bath or a hot shower before bed to relax yourself. Light candles in the bathroom and add a tablespoon of Epsom Salts to your bath water. These will dissolve into your skin and relax you further.

Sleep enhancing environment

Regard your bedroom as a refuge, a place where you go to rest and recover. A refuge where the outside world has no place. Your preparation should include:

- Removing all electronic devices including TVs, tablets and smartphones
- Dimming the light as much as possible. The dimmer the light before you go to bed, the better you will sleep. (Read more about the effects of light.)
- Ensuring that your curtains block out all outside light
- Covering any lights that may emanate from sources such as pilot lights or switches
- Keeping the room cool (below 70°F) ; the warmer the room, the harder it will be to sleep through the night

Electronic devices are a major issue and I believe that you should ban them from your bedroom. Do your TV watching and social networking in another room before you go to sleep. There are apps that can control the kind of light emitted by your computer, tablet or smartphone.

You can also buy amber-coloured glasses that you can wear at night to reduce the blue light falling on your eyes.

Other sleep-enhancing activities

There are things you can do during the day that will enable you to sleep better at night.

- Reduce stress. Read the section on stress again. You must manage your stress to be able to enhance and increase your sleep.
- Get into bright sunlight (when you can); this helps to set your sleep clock
- Do some exercise every day

Light

Exposure to light, particularly blue light, will reduce your urge to sleep. Being in the dark will make you sleepy. As much as possible, try to live like someone who lives without electricity. Follow the natural rhythm of day and night. This natural pattern came to a stop in 1879 when Thomas Edison demonstrated the first practical electrical light bulb at Menlo Park, New Jersey. Today, darkness is optional for most people yet it remains absolutely necessary to our health. Instead of becoming sleepy at night as the light dims, we are bathed in light from a variety of artificial sources. This light keeps us awake and allows us to extend daytime by many hours.

Even the eyes of the blind can 'see' this kind of light, and blind people living in artificially-lit environments end up adopting the same sleep patterns as the sighted people around them. This happens because their sightless eyes still absorb the light that surrounds them.

What this means for your sleep

Now that you know that light keeps you awake and darkness makes you sleepy, you can use this knowledge to modify your behaviour and your environment in order to sleep better.

Daylight

Most of us don't get sufficient exposure to bright sunlight. To sleep better at night, spend some time in bright sunlight whenever you can. Sunlight bathes your eyes in blue light which will help to set your wake/sleep clock and directly affect your ability to sleep better at night.

Get into the sun whenever you can; aim for 20 to 60 minutes a day of direct sunlight. Spend your lunch hour outdoors if possible. Make an effort to be outdoors on a frequent basis; it will help you sleep and lower your stress levels.

Strategies for avoiding light at night

At night, you need to reduce your exposure to blue light which will keep you awake. As discussed earlier, dimming the lights in your home helps. Switch off any lighting that you can practically do. Dim bright lights by fitting dimmer switches where possible, or remove bright light bulbs and replace them with dimmer alternatives.

TVs, tablets, cellphones and computers emit blue light and are major sleep-stealing culprits. There is a well-known app for computers and some smartphones called f.lux which auto-adjusts screens to reduce blue light emissions at night. This works really well and I strongly recommend that you install f.lux or a similar app on all devices that you use at night. (Note: Apple iPhones have had an issue with f.lux in the past; newer IOS releases support this kind of functionality as part of the phone settings.) There are a number of similar apps for other makes of smartphones, like Twilight or Lux Auto Brightness for Android.

Melatonin

Melatonin is a hormone that helps to regulate sleep. It is also involved in other important functions including the regulation of blood pressure.

You can help normalise your melatonin levels by regulating your light exposure, which lowers melatonin levels during the day and keeps you awake in daylight. As it gets dark, melatonin levels rise, making you sleepy and preparing your brain for sleep. This system worked perfectly for hundreds of thousands of years until Edison gave us the light bulb.

Why is melatonin so important? To start with, it regulates your sleep patterns. It is also involved in gut health, bowel motions, and it affects your mood and stress levels. Regulating your melatonin levels will help you in many ways.

Regulating your melatonin levels

Blue light suppresses melatonin. The level of suppression is proportional to the intensity of the light and to the exposure time. Melatonin is made from serotonin, the 'feel good' hormone. Raising your serotonin levels makes you happy, while raising your melatonin levels makes you sleepy.

You get happy when you sleep properly. This is because a regular sleep/wake cycle will naturally increase your levels of serotonin and melatonin, which boost your health and your outlook on life immensely.

Melatonin supplements

If you cannot raise your levels naturally, a melatonin supplement may be a solution. This is not a sleeping pill as it simply signals your body to prepare for sleep. However, it is also a hormone and taking high doses can have consequences. Melatonin is used to treat sleep-related conditions like insomnia and jet lag. Doctors sometimes use melatonin supplements to treat depression-related disorders.

In the right circumstances, taking a melatonin supplement will make you feel drowsy and will help you to fall asleep. There are two different types of supplements: single dose and timed release. Some specialists believe that a slow release of melatonin during the night prolongs sleep. Try this only after you have some experience using the normal release kind.

A short course of melatonin can help to regulate your sleeping patterns but long-term use can be harmful to your health as it has negative effects on the gut lining, which you definitely need to avoid.

Things to bear in mind when you take a melatonin supplement:

- You may need a doctor's prescription for melatonin

- Dosage is critical. Less is better than more. Most supplements are between 3 and 5 mg, which is too much to start with. Break a 3 mg pill into four pieces if you have to. Don't start out taking a dose that is any higher than 1 mg per night. In fact, try 0.5 mg to start with if you can.

- Timing is critical. Never take melatonin during the day. Take your supplement an hour before bedtime.

- The effect is only active for 30 minutes. This means that you need to get to sleep quickly so you must make sure that you are in bed with the lights off and ready to leave for dreamland no more than an hour after you have taken the melatonin.

- Take your melatonin course only for short periods. While there is no fixed course duration, never think of it as a long-term treatment. I would suggest that you take a two or three week course and then stop.

If you wake up and then can't get back to sleep at night, there is a trick that you can try using melatonin which I describe in the next section.

Getting back to sleep

I bet you have had some MOTN. Not in the way it's tagged in Urban Dictionary as an acronym for 'milk running out of the nose'. In our less exotic context, it's something that happens to all of us at some time or another.

Middle Of The Night insomnia (MOTN) is the most common type of insomnia. It affects more than one in three Americans, waking them on at least three nights a week.

Waking up is not the problem; getting back to sleep is the issue. Many of us wake up and then simply cannot get back to sleep. One solution is to take a pill and of course big pharma, who would never miss an opportunity for a revenue stream, has a medication made specifically for MOTN, called Intermezzo.

I don't think that medication has any place in your sleep. While it can be difficult to break out of a long pattern of MOTN, with some patience it can be done naturally.

Before trying to find ways of getting back to sleep, consider some method of preventing the act of waking up in the first place. Here are some to consider:

Reasons for waking up

- Alcohol before bedtime. Limit your alcohol intake at nights and don't drink at all two hours before you go to bed as alcohol can cause MOTN.

- Pets on your bed. Pets can wake you in ways that may not be obvious by making movements, noises or smells. If you have MOTN, do yourself a favour and find your pet a spot on the floor.

- Acid reflux is a common cause of sleep disturbances. A different sleeping position may help. Try sleeping with your upper body elevated. Sometimes losing some weight can help.

- Medication and supplements. If you take these before bedtime, try to vary the time to see if this helps you to sleep better.

- Depression is a common cause of broken sleep. You may not feel depressed, yet your depression may manifest as MOTN.

- Joint and arthritis pain can often cause MOTN. If you have this kind of pain, try taking your pain medication at night, closer to bedtime, and see how this affects your sleep.

- Noisy sleep environment. Noises can wake you; if this happens to you, try to find ways to reduce the noise if you can.

What to do once you're awake

Once it has happened and your eyes pop open in the middle of the night, what can you do about it? Here are some workable options that will definitely help:

- The first rule is, don't switch on the light and don't move! Staying as still as possible in the dark will prevent your mind and body from getting those 'let's get up' signals.

- Stop watching the clock. Marking off the minutes only heightens the stress of not being able to get back to sleep.

- Try relaxing your body to help you fall asleep. Start by tensing and then relaxing your toes. Then tense and relax your ankles and slowly work your way up your body. Feel each part become loose and heavy.

- Once you are relaxed, try to breathe as slowly and shallowly as you can. (See more about Buteyko breathing in the section on Stress – Controlled Breathing). Breathe as if you are not breathing; this will lower your heart rate and blood pressure, which in turn will relax you even more.

- Now fix your thoughts, which may still be racing. Meditate (if you know how to) or else try counting down from 100 and, as soon as a thought interrupts your count, stop counting and start again at 100. Counting has the amazing effect of preventing the mind from dwelling on repetitive thoughts.

Melatonin hack: This trick is worth trying occasionally if you can't get back to sleep using the natural methods above. Take a small dose (about 0.5 mg) of sub-lingual melatonin, a special fast-acting formulation designed to be placed under the tongue for quick absorption. Because it reaches the blood stream quickly, it will deliver a burst of melatonin that will put you to sleep within 10 to 20 minutes.

If all else fails, read this book; it shouldn't take long for you to fall asleep again!

A little MOTN prevention goes a long way

This type of sleeping difficulty can be caused or worsened by your behaviour during the day.

Some of the activities that can affect the duration of your sleep are:

- Naps. If you have difficulty sleeping at night, avoid taking naps during the day
- Don't fall asleep on the couch watching TV
- Don't eat two or three hours before bed
- Get rid of your sleeping pills. All they really do is put you to sleep more quickly but the payback is that they do nothing for the quality or duration of your sleep
- **Recent anecdotal evidence shows that intermittent fasting can improve sleep**

Sleep apps

There are various apps for computers, tablets and smartphones designed to help you have a good night's sleep. They are useful if you are struggling to get to sleep and some can also be used to monitor and document your sleep hours. Some of these apps are free and others are available at a small cost.

Sleep enablers

These apps use gentle sounds, poems and music to relax you in bed and then hopefully send you off to dreamland. Unless otherwise stated, apps are for both Android and iPhone.

*   Relax & Sleep Well, by Glenn Harrold:
    iTunes – http://j.mp/1E9SQPT

*   Sleep Genius – http://j.mp/1CsSiCy

*   Yoga for Insomnia:
    iTunes – http://j.mp/1BtB82V
    Android – http://j.mp/1F0tX71

*   Deep Sleep, with Andrew Johnson – http://j.mp/19XYpEv

*   Insomnia Cure – Sleep Now, with Max Kirsten:
    iTunes – http://j.mp/1HQPmTM

*   Free Relaxing Nature Scenes to Reduce Stress & Anxiety:
    iTunes: http://j.mp/1NiHoTz

Sleep trackers

Rather than help you get to sleep, sleep trackers measure your heart and respiration rates as you sleep. By combining these readings with sleep time, periods of restlessness and sleep cycles, they provide insightful analysis with a sleep time-log. Most sleep tracking apps work in conjunction with a skin sensor that connects to your smartphone. Sensors are often wristbands but there are some under-sheet models. Some of these apps also include a wake-up function.

- Jawbone Up (wrist sensor) – http://j.mp/1yICmNt

- FitBit (wrist and other wearable sensors) – http://j.mp/1HUpLcE

- Beddit (under-sheet) – http://j.mp/1NlvfNR

- SleepTime (no sensor – uses built-in motion tracker) – http://j.mp/1GyBMTf

- SleepBot (no sensor – uses built-in motion tracker) – http://j.mp/1I2aIj0

CHAPTER 20

MOVE

'Life is like riding a bicycle, to keep your balance,
you must keep moving.'

Albert Einstein

We all need to move to survive yet many find it difficult to achieve a balance between moving and not moving at all. On one side, we have people who exercise incessantly and on the other, those who only move to change chairs. In reality, what works best is something in between these extremes.

I believe that there are three essential areas of movement that are directly associated with proper health and longevity. A balance between these areas will allow for a long and healthy life.

It is essential to:

1. Sit less
2. Walk more
3. Exercise occasionally (at a reasonably high intensity)

Paying each of these areas some attention will greatly benefit your health.

Balance

In addition to the three essential body movements, balance is one other crucial area that needs attention. Falls are the most common cause of death by accident for anyone older than 65. In fact, some authorities claim that falls are probably the leading cause of death overall in people over 65. This is because many deaths from conditions unrelated to falling are caused indirectly by an initial fall. For example, a death officially listed as pneumonia can be as a result of a fall that left the patient bedridden, which then caused the pneumonia.

You can find out more about one of the most effective ways to stay alive in the chapter on body balance.

Are you inactive?

The World Health Organization recognises inactivity as the fourth largest cause of death among adults worldwide. A pile of medical studies underscores why this happens. Lack of movement affects your health in many ways, including:

- Heart and blood pressure issues
- Brittle bones
- Obesity
- Diabetes
- Increased risk of cancer, particularly breast and colon cancer
- Depression

Need some motivation to get moving?

Did you know that there is a proven cost-free measure that will reduce the risk of breast cancer in women by more than 50%?

It's called exercise; it costs nothing and you don't have to do a lot of it to get this amazing benefit. A 30-year study that followed over 14,000 women between 1970 and 2001 showed this clearly; so if you are inactive read on!

Raising your activity levels just a little will make a significant difference to your health. You don't have to run a marathon, cycle 100 miles or build big muscles. Just get moving!

Make the time

'I don't have the time.' That's the standard song that most exercise-avoiders sing. If something is important to you, you will find the time. I can assure you that activity is important to you.

Get creative with your time management and you will find a way to make the time. Some of my patients insist that they cannot find a gap to exercise during the week, to which I reply "And what of the weekends?" That leaves the lowest common denominator at two days a week minimum for almost everyone.

Sitting is the new smoking

'My idea of exercise is a good brisk sit.'
Phyllis Diller

As innocuous as it seems, sitting is actually one of the most dangerous activities of daily life and sitting less is a health priority.

The longer you sit without standing up, the worse it is for your health.

Research tells us that office workers spend an average of 10 hours a day perched on their butts. The damage is cumulative and, just in case you think you can diminish your sitting risks by going to the gym at the end of a day of sitting, it has been shown that an hour-a-day workout does not completely mitigate against the risks of spending the rest of the day sitting. In fact, a recent medical study showed that standing three times an hour is better than 30 minutes in the gym.

Sitting makes you old

A key comparison between sitting and the weightlessness experienced by astronauts was made by Dr Joan Vernikos during her time at NASA. She confirmed that astronauts aged about 10 times faster when weightless, compared with the time they spent under the earth's gravity. She then went on to connect the effects of weightlessness to the similar but less dramatic effects of prolonged sitting, eventually writing a book entitled *Sitting Kills, Moving Heals.*

Stand up!

Be conscious of this risk and don't sit for too long. Fixing this is easy. All you have to do is stand up once every 15 to 20 minutes. Nothing else is required. You don't have to run up and down flights of stairs, jog on the spot or do squats.

Just stand up! You can stretch or walk around your desk if you want but that is all that is necessary. If you need help remembering to stand up regularly, there are a number of timer apps that will allow you to set an interval to remind you to do so.

WALKING

> *'Walking is man's best medicine.'*
>
> *Hippocrates*

Walking is the easiest and most effective modification you can make to your lifestyle.

We come from a hundred thousand generations of walkers and as a result, walking is built into our wiring. Dan Lieberman, a Professor of Biological Science at Harvard University, estimates that the average hunter-gatherer walked 10 to 15 kilometres a day. It's not like that today. We have little reason to walk; our work-days are filled by clicking mice and we walk only to answer the call of nature. When we get home, we sit some more as we eat, swipe digital devices and watch TV.

Walking is so accessible; you don't need special shoes or a specialised environment to get started. All you need to do is to make up your mind and walk. Set aside some time to walk; early mornings are a good time and a weekend walk should be part of your chill-out routine.

Make walking your mission

It is easy to increase the distance you walk daily by adding small, unobtrusive extra distances to your normal routine.

Here are some examples:

- Park further from your destination
- Shopping centres are a great way to walk long distances
- Take the long way to your desk or to the toilet
- Walk wherever you can

- Use the stairs instead of the lift
- Get a step tracker (see below)

Starting out

If you are starting a walking program as a former couch potato, start small and don't set big goals. Just walk a little and then rest. Be in the moment, enjoy the scenery, take notice of your surroundings. Don't focus internally on any aches and pains you might have. Don't give up; stick at it and try your best to be mindful and feel the joy of moving your body. Over time, your distance and enjoyment will increase.

If you can, find a walking partner. Talking and walking go well together and your companion will keep you going when your motivation wanes. Do some research; there may be a walking group club you can join in your area.

My walk to freedom

I started walking when I was 30 kg overweight and my knees were so damaged that I couldn't climb a flight of steps. For me, taking the first step was the hardest part and I procrastinated for weeks before taking my first walk around the block. My legs burned all the way and my aches and pains lasted for days. It took me a lot longer than I expected to get walking-fit, and even longer for my body to start feeling the effects and benefits. It took more than a year before I was able to walk distances without effort, but it was worth it in the end!

What gets measured gets done

In my experience, the best motivation to walk more and keep walking is a step-counter. Measuring your steps allows you to initially see how little you actually walk, which may surprise you! Once you get used to walking, your counter will enable you to measure your progress, which often serves as encouragement to keep going.

A step count of 10,000 a day is a good target. You may find that your daily step count is a lot less than that but if you incorporate a short morning or evening walk into your day, this will become much easier to achieve.

There are many ways to count your steps. You can buy a dedicated device like a FitBit, Jawbone or similar but even a manual step counter will do. Another route is to a load a step-tracker app onto your smartphone. These apps work well but they will decrease your battery life. I use Moves on my phone; it does a great job of tracking steps, runs and cycles. Moves also connects to my Medical Aid (as do some other devices), which means that I get health credits for my daily step count.

High intensity walking

When you reach a stage of being able to walk regularly at a steady pace, you can enhance the benefits of your walking by adding some interval training to your walks. An interval is simply a period of faster walking spaced between periods of walking at normal speed.

Dr Hiroshi Nose, of Shinshu University Medical School in Japan, has tested the health benefits of interval walking versus steady pace walking. He split his test subjects into two groups. The interval group employed five cycles of fast, hard walking for three minutes followed by three minutes of strolling. The stroller group ambled along for the entire period. When tested three months later, the stroller group showed almost no improvement in fitness levels, leg strength and blood pressure levels. The interval group, however, showed significant improvements in all these areas.

The take-home message is not to habitually stroll. Occasionally add some intensity to parts of your walks, striding fast enough to ensure that you become out of breath. Use Doctor Nose's method to structure your walks with intervals of hard and easy walking.

EXERCISE

'Exercise, the poor man's plastic surgery.'
Gym poster

The medical literature unanimously agrees that exercise is good for you. People who exercise regularly are healthier and live longer than those who don't.

Less is more

After being involved in fitness training for almost 25 years, I have come to believe that short, high-intensity training sessions build the best overall fitness for any type of activity as opposed to the 'long, slow distance adage'. This applies to any activity and at just about any level.

While some activities lend themselves to long, slow sessions that may be therapeutic for stress, I believe that as a general rule they waste a tremendous amount of time for little return.

But beware of over-exercising; too much exercise causes stress and raises cortisol levels. Don't be one of those people who become addicted to their exercise routines and insert the phrase 'have to' into all their activities.

The message is: irrespective of the type of exercise, choose shorter, more intense exercise sessions over longer efforts. Short, high-intensity work has a much higher return on investment in terms of time and fitness.

29 minutes – proof that less is more

Towards the end of each year there is a cycle race in Johannesburg called the 94.7. Driven indoors by heavy traffic volumes in the city, many cyclists train for the race using stationary bikes in the gym. Last year, I struck up a conversation with two family men who had limited time to train on the road and were riding two-hour sessions in the gym to prepare. After a few heated chats in the sauna, I managed to convince them to reduce their long sessions to 25-minute, high-intensity sessions. As a result, they both rode their fastest race ever; one finishing 20 minutes faster than his best ride in 12 years and the other cutting nine minutes off his best time.

Proof enough for me that less is more.

Aerobic and resistance training

Broadly speaking, there are two types of exercise activities:

- Aerobic exercise; the type of activity you can do for long periods
- Resistance exercise; the type of activity that moves against weight, which can include moving your own body weight as well as making use of various kinds of equipment

Both types of exercise have benefits, but if I had to choose one, I would pick resistance training which I believe, after walking, is the most important exercise you can do. This is the opposite of what most people would choose.

RESISTANCE TRAINING

'Pain is just weakness leaving the body.'
Bodybuilding t-shirt

I find it hard to convince patients and people I talk to that they need to do 'weights'. Many react with disbelief, some stop listening. A common response, particularly from women, is: 'I don't want to get big!' Of course, for most males, 'getting big' is part of the standard male lexicon along with getting laid and getting rich. This area of male fantasy aside, I cannot stress enough the importance of a weekly resistance training session for men and women alike.

Regular resistance training will:

- Reduce the rate at which you age
- Help to retain or rebuild muscle mass that is vital for the immune system
- Make you look better

There are many different ways to resistance-train and I am sure that you will find a method that suits you. Consider employing a personal trainer for a few months to ensure that you do exercises using the correct techniques and to make you feel more comfortable in the weight room.

Routines you can do at home

Body weight training

This kind of resistance exercise can be done pretty much anywhere and is based on your own bodyweight.

Remember, as with any exercise routine, warm up first by walking or jogging lightly for five to ten minutes. Start any exercise slowly and work your way upward in terms of speed, the number of repetitions and the number of sets. Start with a single set and add more sets as you get stronger.

Here are some good ones to get you started:

Squats: Stand straight with your feet shoulder-width wide, feet pointing slightly outward. Keeping your back straight and your hands held out in front of you, slowly lower your butt, sinking down as low as you can go. Keep your dips shallow at first, especially if your joints or leg muscles hurt.

Crunches: Lie face-up on the floor, knees raised and bent or, if you are more comfortable, you can leave your feet on the ground. Put your hands behind your head or fold them over your chest. Slowly curl your head up towards your feet. Keep your neck as straight as possible; don't let your chin touch your chest. Squeeze your abdominal muscles when your head is as far forward as you can manage. Then release and uncurl gently backwards until your back touches the floor again.

Push-ups: Push-ups can be hard to do at first. If you find them too difficult, you can rest your lower body on your knees to make them easier. Lie face down on the floor, while positioning your hands, palms down in front of your shoulders. Push yourself upwards with your hands. At the same time, breathe out and try to keep your body as straight as possible. Lower yourself down until you touch the floor again. Keeping your hands closer to your body makes it easier.

Pull-Ups: Ideally, you need a pull-up bar but often a door lintel will work just as well. To do a pull-up, stand beneath the bar with your feet together. Hold your hands up, palms forward and reach for the bar. Keeping a tight grip, slowly bend your knees and allow your hands to take your full weight. Then slowly pull yourself upward. Once you are as high as you can get, lower yourself slowly again and repeat if you can. Pull-ups are hard so don't get discouraged. You can start by just hanging and then over time, slowly lifting more and more of your body weight. Standing on a small box will also make it easier in the beginning.

You can use YouTube to source and watch professionals doing these routines. You will also be able to find other exercises that you may enjoy doing.

Here are some examples:

*   10 best beginner body weight work-outs:
    http://j.mp/1OgWlae

*   Bodyweight exercises for absolute beginners:
    http://bit.ly/1CGV09x

Gym routines

Weight machines and free weights

This kind of equipment is usually found in the depths of the weights' section of your gym.

I am going to teach you a simple and safe high-intensity routine that I advise beginners and all people who push weights to use to get strong and healthy. The routine is derived from the work of Dr Doug McGuff, an Emergency Medicine physician with a passion for exercise science. Dr McGuff suggests that only a weekly, single-set, high-intensity weight work-out is required to build strength and maintain muscle mass.

Done properly, this routine takes about 20 minutes in the gym including a warm-up.

The main aim is to work at high intensity and induce a deep level of muscle fatigue. This kind of short, sharp stress signals your system to grow and respond in a similar way to the effects of a 'fight or flight' situation. When you start doing this routine, any work you do will feel intense, so you need to increase the weights you use as you become more accustomed to it.

Five movements make up the main routine:

- A push away from the body
- A pull toward the body
- A pull down from the head to shoulder level
- A push upward above the head
- A leg extension

If you feel you can use more, you can add one or two more exercises but sticking to just these five movements will net you 90% of your gains.

How it's done:

- The routine is designed to be done once a week or no more than once every five days (never do back-to-back high intensity days)

- Keep a note of the weight you use for each exercise. This is important, because it gives a progress history and serves as a reminder of how much resistance you need to set on each machine.

- Warm up using a weight light enough that you can do 20 repetitions, thus getting the feel of the movement.

- Load the resistance so that you can do a single set of between 8 to 12 repetitions.

- The slower you do the movement the better. Slower speeds almost entirely eliminate the potential for injury. Never jerk the weights.

- If you cannot manage up to 8 reps, your resistance is too high.

- If you can do more than 12 reps, your resistance is too low.

THE GOAL for each set is to go as hard as you can. Knowing that you have just a single set to do makes it easier to go all out. Failure to complete your last rep, no matter how hard you try, triggers an ancient metabolic mechanism that:

- Sucks glucose from your blood into your muscle cells
- Releases stored fat
- Increases insulin sensitivity
- Raises hormone levels, particularly growth hormone (HGH)
- Releases active substances called myokines that send positive signals to other parts of the body

You can learn more about Dr McGuff's research and his high intensity weight routine here: http://j.mp/1bkvESJ.

Kettlebells

I'm a kettlebell fan. They are amazingly versatile and you can make a home weight room with two or three of them. Kettlebells originated from Russia a few hundred years ago and have been used for training in the Soviet army. They have recently become more popular and are used widely in gyms and homes today.

The ballistic movements you can do with a kettlebell build body strength and suppleness. Kettlebell movements mimic real-world movements better than static weight equipment. A kettlebell work-out will strengthen your back, legs and shoulders. Go slowly if you have a bad back.

Start with a light bell while you get the hang of it. This also allows time for your muscles and joints to become accustomed to the work.

I think the best way to learn how to use kettlebells is by example. If you don't have access to an instructor, there is a selection of beginner work-outs you can watch on YouTube.

Here are some good videos to get you started:

- Kettlebell work-out for beginners – Invade London (this is a fun one): http://j.mp/1Ohm3LN

- Kettlebell work-outs – beginners work-out (good, all-round beginner's routine): http://j.mp/1C8DLfc

- Fitness blender's beginner kettlebell work-out (slightly more advanced): http://j.mp/1xK0Gbu

Good luck and have fun!

Aerobic training

Also called 'cardio', aerobic is a fancy name for any kind of low-to-middle-intensity exercise that does not cause you to get out of breath. My cycling coach explained it best: 'You're aerobic for as long as you can talk; when you start to gasp between words, you're out of the aerobic zone'.

Trained athletes can seemingly go forever doing aerobic exercise. Marathon runners run 100-milers and 24-hour events. The major triathlon events, most of which are heavily oversubscribed, have waiting lists of masochists, champing at the bit to compete in an event comprised of a 4 km swim, followed by a 180 km bicycle ride, topped off with a 42 km run.

But just because some humans can be aerobically active for these types of efforts, it does not mean that it is good for you. A number of studies have highlighted the dangers of too much exercise. You need to strike a balance based on your capabilities, your motivation level and the time available to you.

Getting started

If you are embarking on an exercise programme for the first time or after a long break, start slowly. Less is better than more. I have seen many over-enthusiastic beginners go all out before they are ready, only to hurt themselves and then give up completely.

A gentle walking program is a good place to start (see the section on walking).

Consider a coach

Many beginners find the gym environment to be intimidating. Getting yourself a coach is a good way for you to get yourself into the gym with a professional to guide you. Your coach will also help you to set up a program that is tailored to your capabilities. Coaching can provide guidance that will ensure you improve over time. Missing gym is much harder when you have a pre-booked session with your coach that you are committed to paying for. This kind of pressure will help to ensure that your exercise patterns become regular.

Lastly, don't get married to your coach. Once you have found your feet in the gym, consider going solo or even better, get yourself a training partner.

What not to do – obsession

Once you get going, don't go crazy and become obsessive about timing yourself or competing with others. While a little competition is good, it is all too easy to become addicted to exercise and the competitiveness around it. Remember that you are exercising to be active, to improve your health and to lower your stress levels. Always, always enjoy what you're doing.

What not to do – eat popcorn

The treadmills in my gym are super-advanced and lack only one accessory – a popcorn holder. I say this because so many gym bunnies seem to spend their time on the machines watching TV or talking while moving at the pace of a tortoise. It turns the activity into a standing-up movie experience, lacking only the popcorn to munch.

When you do an activity, be there mentally. Try things like varying your pace and increasing and decreasing resistance levels to make your exercise more challenging and engaging. Also, look at your form and try to improve the way you do your exercise. Good form helps to ensure that you do not do repetitive movements that could injure you in the long term. Ask for some assistance or try to mimic the actions of someone who is visibly doing a more professional job of the exercise. The staff walking around the gym are there to help you so don't be scared to approach them.

Some varieties to consider

The treadmill is the most popular piece of gym equipment. While most gyms have more treadmills than any other type of exercise equipment, there are many alternatives. Here are some of my recommendations:

Rowing machine: To me, rowing is the best all-round activity you can do in a gym. When done properly, rowing will give you a whole-body work-out. It is also quite easy to vary the intensity of your work-out as you row and hard rowing can make you breathless in minutes. The only downside is that to row properly requires some practice. Try to get a rower or a coach with some rowing experience to give you a lesson when you begin.

Elliptical walker: This can give a good, almost-total body work-out when used with arm and leg movement. Because it supports body weight, it is often good for people with leg and knee issues. If you try hard, you can really tax your body on one of these.

Stationary bike: Great for any level or size of exerciser. Your set-up on the bike is important, so get help when you start. Incorrect settings can lead to a painful ride or knee and hip injuries. If your butt hurts when you ride, get someone to check your set-up so that your ride is more comfortable.

Here is a list of some of the aerobic exercise activities you can do.

Outdoors:

- Walking or running
- Cycling
- Rowing
- Skiing
- Swimming

Indoors:

- Running/walking on a treadmill
- Stair climbing
- Rowing machine
- Stationary bicycle
- Elliptical trainer
- Indoor swimming

CHAPTER 21

BODY BALANCE

In earlier chapters we addressed mental balance; now let's have a quick look at body balance. This is an extremely important yet rarely practised skill.

As we age, our ability to balance declines. This translates into an increased potential for falls and spills as we get older. It is true that the older you are the harder you fall. So much so, that falls are the probable leading cause of death in people older than 65.

Your potential for falling will increase as you get more active so it makes sense to spend a little time every week working on your body balance.

Balancing methods

There are a number of ways in which to strengthen your body balance. Here are the basic exercises you need to do. Once you have mastered these, you can increase the difficulty and improve your results by doing these same exercises on a Power Plate machine or using a stability ball or a half-sphere ball. You can also take up Pilates or yoga.

All the exercises below are done using a chair, for safety. Once you become more confident, they can be done without it.

1) Single leg balance

- Place a chair within reaching distance in case you need to hold it to keep your balance
- Stand with your feet together and your arms at your sides
- Lift one leg and balance on the other
- Hold this pose for between 10 and 20 seconds
- Lower the leg and repeat for the other leg
- Repeat the exercise 5–10 times

2) Clock balance

- Stand on your right leg with your hand on a chair placed on your right side
- Keep your head still and look straight ahead
- Hold your left hand out at the 12 o'clock position, directly in front of you, palm down and parallel to the floor
- Keeping your left leg as still as possible, with your outstretched arm parallel to the floor, sweep your arm to the 3 o'clock position
- Bring it back to the 12 o'clock position
- Then try and sweep it all the way back to your 6 o'clock, almost behind you
- Repeat these moves 5–10 times
- Move the chair to your left side and repeat the exercise

3) Arm-up and leg-out

- Stand on your right leg with your hand on a chair placed on your right
- Keeping your body as straight as possible, raise your left arm
- Raise your left leg off the floor
- Hold the position for 10 to 20 seconds
- Repeat the exercise 5–10 times
- Move the chair to your left side and repeat the exercise

There are many more variations. Use YouTube to search for some examples.

Here is a good one:

Balance training exercises: http://j.mp/1bkGYOl

My body un-balance

A while back, I was having coffee with some friends when one of them, Shaun, mentioned that his doctor had tested his ability to stand on one leg. "Why on earth would she do that?" I asked. Shaun didn't answer my question but simply said "You try". To my surprise, and to the enjoyment of the group, I couldn't balance for more than a few seconds.

I resolved to become more balanced. The act of putting my shoes on became the daily tool I used. No longer did I put my shoes on while seated; I would only allow myself to do this standing up. It was initially a fiasco because I needed a wall behind me to balance against and so took me much longer than usual. However, over the next few months it became easier and I can now do it quite effortlessly.

Last week, while cleaning up around our patio, my foot became wedged between two objects, almost causing me to fall over. Without my improved balance, I am certain that I would have fallen sideways, my foot trapped, and I would have undoubtedly broken my ankle.

The message here is that you should look at using simple strategies to slowly improve your balance.

CHAPTER 21

GROWING MUSCLE LEGALLY

'Sweat dries; blood clots; bones heal. Suck it up princess!'
Broscience 101

The quote above sums up the attitude of some of the men and women who spend their time in the gym trying to grow muscle. They will take any kind of medication or potion that enables them to 'get bigger'; this includes any combination of growth hormone, steroids, insulin, testosterone plus many lesser-known medications. They also indulge in rituals that dictate the times and quantities of the supplements they drink and the food they eat. Health goes by the wayside in the quest for muscle gain.

If I had a dollar for every time I have been approached for a sure-fire method to gain muscle, I would be writing this from the deck of my yacht in the Mediterranean. However, the insulin hypothesis that is central to this book, which aims to reduce average insulin levels allowing for weight loss and a reduction in various dread diseases, can theoretically also be used to grow muscle.

The realisation that body builders use insulin to grow muscle came to me when I noticed one of the big body-building heavies rummaging around in a garbage bin in our gym change room. I was surprised to find that the medicine vial that had been secreted in the trash for him to collect was commercial insulin. My subsequent insulin research has led me to believe that the correct stimulation, after a period of intermittent fasting, may well induce the body to produce a good surge of insulin naturally, without having to resort to injections.

Hence this programme, which is aimed at growing muscle and increasing fat burning.

Here's how it's done

First, you need to become used to intermittent fasting. Ideally, if you have weight to lose, then you need to have fasted for a long enough time for you to have lost at least half of your targeted weight. The reason for this is that you need to be as insulin-sensitive as possible for the plan to work and you will not be that sensitive if you are carrying too much weight. If you are lucky enough not to have any significant weight to lose, you can start as soon as you can manage a 20-hour fast.

Important: The plan is designed to be used once a week only. This is because I suspect that it will become ineffective if used too often and it may also lead to weight gain.

Requirements: You will need a good protein shake that is high in BCAAs. The shake you choose will work better if it contains a little sugar; do not use a low-sugar shake that has artificial sweeteners. When preparing your shake, use the recommended dose and mix it either with milk or water. If you can tolerate it, milk is preferable because it adds to the available BCAAs and protein.

Optional requirement: Access to a sauna after the work-out is complete is a bonus. A 10- or 15-minute sauna after your routine will raise growth hormone levels, as has been shown in a number of studies. This growth hormone rise will support and encourage muscle growth as well as fat burning.

1. Fast for 20 hours; try to be as strict as possible during this period.

2. Drink your shake when you get to the gym; try to finish as much of the shake as you can in one go. Thereafter drink water as needed if you are thirsty.

3. Do a hard weights routine, using the heaviest weights that you can safely manage. Use the weight routine I describe in the Resistance Training section of this book as a guideline. The idea is to have a single, all-out weight work-out once a week, rather than a number of almost-all-out routines. It is crucial to make sure that you try as hard as you can without hurting yourself.

What happens

Super-hard muscle contractions release a cascade of signalling proteins (called myokines) that are designed to cause adaptations that enable the body to deal with the increased loads placed on the muscles. These adaptations include muscle growth to handle more weight in the future as well as metabolic changes to allow greater fat burning. This is the reason why it is essential to try as hard as you can. Doing fewer sets at greater intensity ensures that your muscles send the correct signals to make certain that they can grow to handle the load.

Done correctly, this routine will combine the insulin surge caused by the protein shake with the myokine cascade caused by the high-intensity muscle load, allowing for maximum entry of proteins, amino acids and glucose into muscle cells which will spur growth. A sauna after your work-out will also increase the growth hormone spike.

In hormone terms, this work-out can safely simulate the combined effects of an injection containing both growth hormone and insulin.

Ideally, this programme should not be used on a continual basis. It will work best if used for a two or three month period and then repeated again after a rest of a few months. During the 'rest' phase you can use any other programme you choose.

CHAPTER 22

YOU LIE! EAT LESS, EXERCISE MORE

'The only way you get that fat off is to eat less and exercise more.'

Jack LaLanne

Let's try to lay to rest the great 'exercise to lose weight debate' – otherwise known as the 'calories in equal calories out' conundrum – a concept that implies the human body is a simple machine and, in energy terms, it can be treated as such. In other words, it is a machine that uses fuel empirically with an energy usage that can be measured like a car's petrol consumption.

'Eat less and exercise more' is the advice many doctors and weight-loss specialists extend to their patients. This piece of nonsense has been repeated as truth for so long, it was probably carved onto the back of Moses's stone tablets when he descended Mount Sinai.

Unfortunately, when it comes to weight loss, the human body is a lot smarter than a car engine and both parts of this double-barrelled pearl of wisdom work to pave the road to obesity.

One, eating less makes you fat

A few days of eating less is all it takes to send the body an ancient 'famine' signal, which then translates into a metabolic slow-down to mitigate a perceived food shortage. Eating less means eating smaller portions, which translates into continuous calorie restriction. This produces a state of semi-famine, which is completely different to the metabolic state produced by intermittent fasting. The body's response to continuous calorie restriction is to slow down processes that consume energy and to store as much fat as possible. This has been scientifically measured, with some studies showing weight gain in subjects as their daily calorie intake is reduced.

Two, exercising more makes you fat

The more you exercise, the more you eat; it's as simple as that.

Some initial weight loss often occurs when an overweight person first starts to exercise but, over time, this weight loss will stabilise and eventually stop as food intake rises to balance energy output. A quick look at the crowds, dressed in overstretched Lycra, gathering at the start of road or cycle races will quickly reveal how true this is.

But wait! There is a way to exercise yourself thinner.

Read on.

Energy economics primer

The oldest debate in the world of weight loss is whether calories in really equal calories out.

Believe it or not, we can fly ambulance drones equipped with automatic heart defibrillators to rescue heart-attack victims, but the might of science has yet to answer this question in a way that achieves general agreement.

What we do know for sure is:

1. Exercise increases appetite

2. Body fat can only be deposited when there is an overall energy surplus

The body, being a smart machine, responds to exercise by hoarding fuel. As soon as supplies become available, it rushes to replace its muscle and liver glycogen (stored glucose) deposits, after which it will store any excess energy as fat.

This is why it becomes almost impossible not to eat more after exercise. In fact, many people exercise because they think that they can eat more and supposedly not put on weight. But a little extra food quickly makes up for a lot of extra running. After long endurance events, competitors sit down for monster, post-event meals, gorging on all kinds of delicacies that were forbidden before the event and during training.

This, in general, is why most amateur endurance athletes (weekend warriors) are a little tubby.

Let's dig deeper with some basic arithmetic.

Change in body fat = Energy consumed – Energy expended

Which is another way of saying to lose weight, eat less, exercise more, which does not work in practice because food intake goes up to balance the extra output. This means that energy consumption and expenditure are linked. (If you want to dig deeper you can find a brilliant explanation of how they are linked, written by Dr Peter Attia (The Eating Academy) here: http://eatingacademy.com/nutrition/do-calories-matter)

The energy consumed part of the equation above just climbs to meet energy expenditure.

Bear with me, there is a way to fix this!

Daily energy requirements for an average 30-something sedentary man are about 2,400 calories. This increases to about 3,000 calories per day for an active man.

Let's do a thought-experiment to see how this would affect Les, a hypothetical 30-year old man, over the course of a week. Les is an IT specialist who drives to work, where he spends the rest of his day behind a computer monitor; after work, he does the dinner-in-front-of-the-TV thing and then goes to sleep.

Here is how two weeks in Les's life would look, one in couch-potato mode and another where he trains for three days. Each of Les's one-hour gym sessions adds about 400 calories a day to his energy requirements.

Energy requirements: Couch-potato week = 16,800 calories

- 7 days @ 2,400 calories

Energy requirements: With 3 training days = 18,000 calories

- 4 days @ 2,400 calories
- 3 days @ 2,800 calories

Results: Eat less, exercise more

Les, being human, will, whether he realizes it or not, begin to eat more to make up for the extra energy he uses on his active days.

So, while he may not gain weight, he will not lose any weight either.

Results: Three training days plus fasting

Let's assume that Les employs a 20-hour fasting window on his exercise days.

No matter how large his single daily meal becomes, he cannot reasonably eat enough to make up for his daily calorie deficit. Even if he consumes a meal of 1,000 calories, a big meal by any standards, and then adds an after-dinner snack of 500 calories, he would still be about 1,300 calories short of his theoretical daily energy requirements.

Over a week this deficit would then add up to about 3,900 calories less than his theoretical requirements. Even if our Les is little less than disciplined on his non-fasting days, he could still manage to be behind his requirements by between 2,000 and 3,000 calories. This relatively small deficit is the key. It will add up over time and eventually reflect as a slow but significant weight loss.

The take-home message

You can speed up your weight loss by the intelligent use of intermittent fasting combined with exercise!

Practically speaking, as long as you are not overeating on non-fasting days, you can eat as much as you like in your eating window on the days you exercise and still lose weight.

Remember to eat real food and to resist the sugar-and-sweet urge as much as you can; among other ill effects, high sugar loads make you older faster.

CHAPTER 23

A DAY IN THE LIFE

Many people seem to be curious about what I eat and how I get through my days, which I am happy to disclose, but first let me tell you a short story.

Last weekend, just a few days after 2016 New Year, I was using the pull-up bar in my gym, when I noticed a grizzled older gentleman peering quizzically up at me. As I dropped to my feet, he asked the strangest question.

"Are those still your knees?" he said.

"Excuse me…?"

He repeated the question again; I was speechless.

"I'm Dr F. Don't you remember me, I operated on your knees over 20 years ago?" he said, by way of explanation.

"Yes, they are."

"Amazing!" he said. 'I would have sworn that by now you would have had multiple knee replacements."

He had a point. All those years ago, I used to visit him quarterly and he would inject cortisone into both my knees which, at the time, were permanently swollen like hot-air balloons. When the cortisone stopped working, he sent me for a radioactive treatment that was supposed to kill the joint tissue that was causing the swelling. It did, but only worked for a year or so.

Eventually, I gave up on a medical system that seemed intent on pumping me full of meds and found that I could bicycle my knees into submission. As a result, for many years, I used to swallow painkillers every time I rode a bicycle. Today, I take no medications at all and my knees are fine. Today my general health is good and all blood tests for markers of inflammation, which used to be sky high, are now normal.

A normal day – food

During the week, I try not to eat during the daytime. Over weekends, I relax a bit and often walk my dog, Dash, to breakfast on Saturday morning. On these days, I have a three-egg omelette with cheese and mushrooms and some extra avocado on the side.

Thus, most week-days, I get through the day drinking water as often as I need to as well as two or three cups of coffee with a tablespoon of cream. I use no sweeteners.

For dinner, I eat a protein mixed with green salad drizzled liberally with olive oil; some veggies; and the occasional serving of rice or cold potato salad. I usually have a shot of whiskey as well. After dinner, I have green tea and some chocolate but make sure that I don't eat after 9 o'clock at night. I no longer obsess about carbs and, while I would never take sugar directly, I sometimes eat foods that contain it.

When I eat, I don't watch portion sizes and I eat until I am full. Now that I don't officially Bant, I don't mind the occasional bowl of ice-cream or dessert. I also have a pizza every now and then, when the mood strikes me.

A normal day – exercise

I must admit that I gym almost every day, which is not something that I expect from my patients! This is my routine:

- Easy 30 mins walk almost every morning
- One hard weight session a week (25 mins max)
- One high-intensity indoor cycling session a week (25 mins max) and one longer, easy session
- One or two sessions a week on the treadmill (30 to 40 mins)
- One or two sessions a week rowing (20 mins)
- I don't do any stretching because I believe that it's built into the exercise routines
- I don't do specific abdominal work for the same reason
- I try to hang or do pull-ups every second day
- I practise my balance every day; I always stand up to put my shoes on
- I try to sauna or steam bath at least five times a week
- I shower with cold water all year round (winter is very, very hard!)

A normal day – supplements

- 2–3 grams of omega-3 oil
- 5,000 IU vitamin D3
- 100 mg co-enzyme-Q10
- Multi-B vitamin
- Occasional magnesium oil spray on joints or any areas that become sore as a result of exercise
- Psyllium husks – 1 tablespoon in a glass of water on most days

There are so many supplements out there, each with an earnest reason for you to swallow them and why, once you do, they will change your life, cure cancer, deflect bullets and make you immortal. Marketing BS aside, choosing a vitamin or supplement is a difficult decision for anyone standing in the vitamin isle to make; having to choose between price, ingredients and dosages. With this in mind, I try to keep my supplements to a minimum.

My vital vitamin is D3, which I believe at least 90% of all people in the civilized world are deficient of, simply because we don't get enough sunlight. I remember watching a professor of obstetrics and gynaecology give a lecture on YouTube, where she said that she believed breast cancer is largely a disease caused by vitamin D deficiency, which is a frightening statement.

After vitamin D3, I choose omega-3 because we cannot make it ourselves and it is absolutely vital for cell wall integrity. Weak or damaged cell membranes are leaky in both directions and probably predispose to the formation of cancer growths as well as many auto-immune diseases. Omega-3 is almost completely absent from our food supply because any food containing a reasonable amount of omega-3 has no appreciable shelf-life, as it is removed during processing.

I take co-enzyme-Q10 because I am an active old fart and co-enzyme-Q10 levels decline with old age, especially in the heart and muscle mitochondria. The multi-Bs are for methylation and I take the magnesium oil because almost everyone is short of magnesium. For the rest, I hope it comes from the real food that I eat.

For my gut health, I take psyllium husks a few times a week. I try to eat pure butter occasionally, as the butyric acid it contains is the best food for the cells of the intestinal lining. When possible I eat fermented foods, especially sauerkraut and milk kefir and occasionally kombucha tea.

CONCLUSION

'Last time I was sober, man I felt bad,
worst hangover that I ever had.
It took six hamburgers and Scotch all night,
nicotine for breakfast just to put me right.'
Dire Straits

Dear reader, it's your turn.

You can live the Dire Straits way or you can make a few changes. I have done all the heavy lifting, now it's over to you.

You can learn from my mistakes. My initial efforts led me to publish a guidebook, *The Decarb Diet*, in early 2013, introducing the low-carb concept. For a few years afterward, I toed the Banting/LCHF (low-carb, high-fat) line; I counselled patients, gave talks and sang from Noakes' hymnbook. Over time, I realised that the system was imperfect; it worked well for some, partially for others, and not at all for those who needed it most.

I hope that after reading this book I have managed to convince you that Banting or any other diet, low-carb, high-carb or whatever, cannot work unless insulin, the real culprit, is dealt with directly.

You can fix yourself

Spend some time on yourself, reduce your stress levels, bring your body back into balance and allow it to heal itself. Adopt new habits and discard old ones; do it for yourself, it's for a good cause. YOU are a good cause and it can be done.

While we all have non-negotiable habits, habits that we know are not good for us, we also have habits that can be dropped with little consequence and even sometimes with great relief. Make the effort to replace some of your old habits with new, healthier ones.

I know that no-one (who is 'normal') can adopt all the advice in this book. However, by taking a little time and applying some effort, you will be able to work towards a personal recipe that will work for you. The small discomforts that often accompany the changing of habits will be worth the struggle.

From a diet perspective, the book says:

- Beware of fad diets that cut out complete food groups.
- Stop obsessing about carbs; just eat real food.
- Stop obsessing about calories and weighing portions; just eat your fill.
- Stop being a slave to your hunger and the timing of your next meal; just eat when you choose to eat.

Move your body a little more (or less if you're an obsessive exerciser). Sit less and walk more, especially outdoors. Reconnect yourself with nature; feel the drizzle of rain on your face, smell the scents on the breeze, sweat a little. Take your shoes off more often, go barefoot and savour the feel of grass beneath your feet. Get your feet dirty, some sand between your toes, glory in the texture and temperature of the earth as it seeps into your soles.

Reduce your electronic time; take care to be attentive to the people around you; spend time with friends or family; put people before some meaningless Facebook post or tweets from some twats.

In other words, be good to yourself. I want you to live a long, healthy and happy life.

REFERENCES

While the references below are split by chapter in order to make looking them up easier, I have purposely avoided scattering academic-type reference links throughout the book to lend the book less of an academic feel. The references are not exhaustive but I have tried to include the most important ones. No excuses, but there are so many studies to read that a professional medical researcher who spends his whole life reading medical journals recently said that about 200 articles appear daily and in order for him to read them all, he would need them to stop being published for about 100 years just so that he could catch up.

CHAPTER 1: A CIRCUS OF EXPERTS

- A brief history of how breakfast got its 'healthy' rep http://www.huffingtonpost.com/2014/10/06/breakfast-most-important-history_n_5910054.html
- HCFS Consumption http://corn.org/publications/statistics/hfcs-consumption/
- Diamond, J. The worst mistake in the history of the human race. *Discover Magazine*, University of California at Los Angeles, Medical School.
- A new dietary paradigm? Low-carbohydrate and high-fat intake can manage obesity and associated conditions: Occasional survey http://www.samj.org.za/index.php/samj/article/view/7302/5506

CHAPTER 2: WHY BANTING IS BROKEN

- *Banting: A Biography* by Michael Bliss
- Letter on corpulence, addressed to the public
  https://archive.org/details/letteroncorpulen00bant
- Twinkie diet helps nutrition professor lose 27 pounds
  http://edition.cnn.com/2010/HEALTH/11/08/twinkie.diet.
  professor
  Twinkies diet: http://anthonycolpo.com/twinkie-diet-helps-
  nutrition-professor-lose-27-pounds/
- Eats nothing but McDonald's for three months,
  LOSES 37 POUNDS. https://www.youtube.com/user/
  mcdonaldsdietburger
  McDonald's diet: http://newsfeed.time.com/2014/01/05/
  teacher-loses-37-pounds-after-three-month-mcdonalds-
  diet/
- *The Bulletproof Diet* by Dave Asprey
- Top 15 reasons you are not losing weight on a low-carb
  diet. http://authoritynutrition.com/15-reasons-not-losing-
  weight-on-a-low-carb-diet
- Pushing past a plateau. https://www.atkins.com/how-it-
  works/atkins-blogs/colette-heimowitz/pushing-past-a-
  plateau

CHAPTER 3: KNOW YOUR ENEMY, ITS NAME IS INSULIN

- Deaths: Diabetes remains the 7th leading cause of death in
  the United States in 2010
  http://www.diabetes.org/diabetes-basics/statistics/
- Global patterns of cancer incidence and mortality rates and
  trends
  http://cebp.aacrjournals.org/content/19/8/1893/
  F1.expansion.html

CHAPTER 4: DROWNING IN INSULIN

- Alberto Villoldo: Shamanic Biohacker
  https://www.bulletproofexec.com/79-shamanic-
  biohacking-with-alberto-villoldo-podcast
- Albert Schweitzer: http://www.nytimes.com/learning/
  general/onthisday/bday/0114.html
- The discovery of insulin
  http://www.nobelprize.org/educational/medicine/insulin/
  discovery-insulin.html
- Frederick Banting (1891–1941) and Charles Best (1899–1978
  http://www.sciencemuseum.org.uk/broughttolife/people/
  frederickbanting
- Plasma fasting glucose and insulin (GLU_E)
  http://www.cdc.gov/nchs/nhanes/nhanes2007-2008/Glu_E.
  htm
- National Health and Nutrition Examination Survey;
  2007–2008 Data Documentation, Codebook, and
  Frequencies
  http://www.cdc.gov/nchs/nhanes/nhanes2007-2008/Glu_E.
  htm

CHAPTER 5: INSULIN RESISTANCE – BANTING'S MAJOR WEAKNESS

- Mel Gibson interview by Edward Douglas
  www.comingsoon.net – August 13, 2012
- Accord Study – Action to control cardiovascular risk in
  diabetes (ACCORD) trial.
  https://www.nhlbi.nih.gov/health-pro/resources/heart/
  accord-trial

CHAPTER 6: WHY YOU SHOULD FEAR DIABETES

- Insulin use and increased risk of mortality in type 2 diabetes: A cohort study
  http://onlinelibrary.wiley.com/doi/10.1111/j.1463-1326.2009.01125.x/abstract
- Debate: long-term safety of insulin in type 2 diabetes
  https://www.idf.org/sites/default/files/attachments/DV59-1-Debate_EN.pdf
- Increased cancer-related mortality for patients with type 2 diabetes who use sulfonylureas or insulin
  http://care.diabetesjournals.org/content/29/2/254.abstract
- Intensive blood glucose control reduced type 2 diabetes mellitus-related end points
  http://acpjc.acponline.org/Content/130/1/issue/ACPJC-1999-130-1-002.htm

CHAPTER 7: WHY YOU HAVE TO CHECK YOUR BLOOD SUGAR

- Definition and diagnosis of diabetes mellitus and intermediate hyperglycemia
  http://www.who.int/diabetes/publications/Definition%20and%20diagnosis%20of%20diabetes_new.pdf

CHAPTER 8: EXCESS PROTEIN – BANTING'S MAJOR DANGER

- Low protein intake is associated with a major reduction in IGF-1, cancer, and overall mortality in the 65 and younger but not older population – Valter Longo
  http://www.cell.com/cell-metabolism/abstract/S1550-4131(14)00062-X

- Dr Mercola, Dec 2015
  http://articles.mercola.com/sites/articles/
  archive/2015/12/21/excessive-protein-intake.aspx
- Fassano – IGF-1
  http://news.harvard.edu/gazette/1999/04.22/igf1.story.html
- Interview with Valter Longo, IFOM – UCSC Longevity
  Institute
  https://www.youtube.com/watch?v=23tcu7q0DBU
- Controlling protein intake may be key to longevity, studies
  show
  https://www.elsevier.com/connect/controlling-protein-
  intake-may-be-key-to-longevity
- C. elegans
  http://artchester.net/2015/02/healthspan-lifespan-healthy-
  aging/
- Kidney stones: High protein diet brings risk of kidney stones
  http://www.ncbi.nlm.nih.gov/pmc/articles/PMC1169452/

CHAPTER 9: REDUCING INSULIN: THE HARD WAY

- Life after gastric bypass: The surprising real story: 3 sisters, 3
  very different results. Here's what can go right – and wrong
  http://www.prevention.com/weight-loss/weight-loss-tips/
  weight-loss-gastric-bypass-surgery
- Reversal of type 2 diabetes: Normalisation of beta cell
  function in association with decreased pancreas and liver
  triacylglycerol
  http://www.ncbi.nlm.nih.gov/pubmed/21656330
- Endoscopic findings and outcomes of revisional procedures
  in patients with weight recidivism after gastric bypass
  http://www.sages.org/meetings/annual-meeting/abstracts-
  archive/endoscopic-findings-and-outcomes-of-revisional-

procedures-in-patients-with-weight-recidivism-after-gastric-bypass
- Roux en Y gastric bypass: How and why it fails? http://www.omicsonline.org/open-access/roux-en-y-gastric-bypass-how-and-why-it-fails-2161-1076-4-165.pdf

CHAPTER 10: REDUCING INSULIN THE EASY WAY

- Fasting girl https://en.wikipedia.org/wiki/Fasting_girl
- The true stories of 4 Victorian fasting girls http://mentalfloss.com/article/51477/true-stories-4-victorian-fasting-girls
- The Jacob Case http://www.welshlegalhistory.org/research-jacob-trial-report.php
- Sarah Jacobs: The fasting girl http://www.bbc.co.uk/blogs/wales/entries/bd974e20-46c0-3228-8109-3cdc993fa410
- Why fasting is now back in fashion http://www.telegraph.co.uk/lifestyle/11524808/The-history-of-fasting.html
- Features of a successful therapeutic fast of 382 days' duration
- http://www.ncbi.nlm.nih.gov/pmc/articles/PMC2495396/pdf/postmedj00315-0056.pdf

CHAPTER 11: FASTING: BENEFITS & MYTHS

- Diet that mimics fasting appears to slow aging http://news.usc.edu/82959/diet-that-mimics-fasting-appears-to-slow-aging

- Fasting for three days can regenerate entire immune system, study finds
  http://www.telegraph.co.uk/news/uknews/10878625/Fasting-for-three-days-can-regenerate-entire-immune-system-study-finds.html
- Effect of starvation and very low calorie diets on protein-energy interrelationships in lean and obese subjects
  http://archive.unu.edu/unupress/food2/UID07E/UID07E11.HTM
- Drug companies enjoy profits from off-label sales of HGH
  http://www.rightinginjustice.com/news/2012/12/23/drug-companies-enjoy-profits-from-off-label-sales-of-hgh
- Growth hormone deemed illegal for off-label antiaging use
  http://www.medscape.org/viewarticle/515665
- An integrated view of oxidative stress in aging: Basic mechanisms, functional effects, and pathological considerations
  http://ajpregu.physiology.org/content/292/1/R18
- How intermittent fasting stacks up among obesity-related myths, assumptions, and evidence-backed facts
  http://fitness.mercola.com/sites/fitness/archive/2013/03/01/daily-intermittent-fasting.aspx
- Time-restricted feeding is a preventative and therapeutic intervention against diverse nutritional challenges
  http://www.cell.com/cell-metabolism/abstract/S1550-4131%2814%2900498-7
- Free-radical theory of aging
  https://en.wikipedia.org/wiki/Free-radical_theory_of_aging
- Feast then famine – how fasting might make our cells more resilient to stress
  http://theconversation.com/feast-then-famine-how-fasting-might-make-our-cells-more-resilient-to-stress-38808

- Why fasting bolsters brain power: Mark Mattson at TEDxJohnsHopkinsUniversity
  https://www.youtube.com/watch?v=4UkZAwKoCP8
- *The fasting cure* by Upton Sinclair
- Augmented growth hormone (GH) secretory burst frequency and amplitude mediate enhanced GH secretion during a two-day fast in normal men
- http://www.ncbi.nlm.nih.gov/pubmed?Db=pubmed&Cmd=ShowDetailView&TermToSearch=1548337
- Intermittent versus daily calorie restriction: which diet regimen is more effective for weight loss?
  http://www.ncbi.nlm.nih.gov/pubmed/21410865
- Chronic Intermittent Fasting Improves Cognitive Functions and Brain Structures in Mice
  http://www.ncbi.nlm.nih.gov/pmc/articles/PMC3670843/
- Fasting Supercharges Your Brain – Here is How
  http://humansarefree.com/2013/12/fasting-supercharges-your-brain-here-is.html
- Alternate-day fasting in non-obese subjects: effects on body weight, body composition, and energy metabolism
  http://ajcn.nutrition.org/content/81/1/69.full
- The influence of higher protein intake and greater eating frequency on appetite control in overweight and obese men
  http://www.ncbi.nlm.nih.gov/pubmed/20339363
- Biochemistry. 5th edition. Section 30.3Food Intake and Starvation Induce Metabolic Changes
  http://www.ncbi.nlm.nih.gov/books/NBK22414/
- Fasting: The History, Pathophysiology and Complications
  http://www.ncbi.nlm.nih.gov/pmc/articles/PMC1274154/

CHAPTER 12: FOUNDATIONS OF FASTING

- La Comparsita
  https://en.wikipedia.org/wiki/La_cumparsita
- Tango's most famous song
  http://totango.net/cumparsita.html
- A brief history of how breakfast got its 'healthy' rep
  http://www.huffingtonpost.com/2014/10/06/breakfast-
  most-important-history_n_5910054.html

CHAPTER 13: BANTING BEGONE!

- Increased meal frequency does not promote greater weight
  loss in subjects who were prescribed an 8-week equi-
  energetic energy-restricted diet.
  http://www.ncbi.nlm.nih.gov/pubmed/19943985
- Thermogenesis in humans after varying meal time
  frequency.
  http://www.ncbi.nlm.nih.gov/pubmed/3592618

CHAPTER 14: A NEW DEAL

- Lethal algae take over beaches in northern France
  http://www.theguardian.com/world/2009/aug/10/france-
  brittany-coast-seaweed-algae
- Court rules France responsible in toxic algae case
  http://www.dailymail.co.uk/wires/ap/article-2701172/
  Court-rules-France-responsible-toxic-algae-case.html
- Mcdonald's burger looks the same – 14 years later. Time.
  com.
  http://newsfeed.time.com/2013/04/25/mcdonalds-burger-
  looks-the-same-14-years-later/

Water

- Total and specific fluid consumption as determinants of bladder cancer risk
  http://onlinelibrary.wiley.com/doi/10.1002/ijc.21587/abstract
- Over 300 pollutants in U.S. tap water
  http://www.ewg.org/tap-water
- Centers for Disease Control and Prevention – 2012 CDC Water Fluoridation Statistics
  http://www.cdc.gov/fluoridation/statistics/2012stats.htm

Meat

- Why processed meat is bad for you
  http://authoritynutrition.com/why-processed-meat-is-bad/
- Hogging it; estimates of antimicrobial abuse in livestock
  http://www.iatp.org/files/Hogging_It_Estimates_of_Antimicrobial_Abuse_in.pdf

Poultry

- Chicken more popular than beef in U.S. for first time in 100 years
  http://www.huffingtonpost.com/2014/01/02/chicken-vs-beef_n_4525366.html

- Arsenic-based animal drugs and poultry
  http://www.fda.gov/AnimalVeterinary/SafetyHealth/ProductSafetyInformation/ucm257540.htm

- Summary report of poultry imports report for December 2015
  http://www.sapoultry.co.za/pdf-statistics/summary-imports-report.pdf

- Bovine Somatotropin (BST)
  http://www.fda.gov/AnimalVeterinary/SafetyHealth/
  ProductSafetyInformation/ucm055435.htm

Fish

- Farm-raised salmon poisoned with petrochemicals
  http://www.naturalhealth365.com/0890_farm_raised_
  salmon.html

- Seafood selector
  http://seafood.edf.org

Sugar and fructose

- Uric acid and hypertension: Cause or effect? (2010)
  http://www.ncbi.nlm.nih.gov/pubmed/20425019

- Pediatric nonalcoholic fatty liver disease
  http://contemporarypediatrics.modernmedicine.com/
  contemporary-pediatrics/content/tags/biomarker/
  pediatric-nonalcoholic-fatty-liver-disease

- Consumption of honey, sucrose, and high-fructose corn
  syrup produces similar metabolic effects in glucose-tolerant
  and -intolerant individuals
  http://jn.nutrition.org/content/early/2015/09/02/
  jn.115.218016.abstract

Sweeteners

- Sugar substitutes – what's safe and what's not
  http://articles.mercola.com/sites/articles/
  archive/2013/10/07/sugar-substitutes.aspx

- Consumption of artificial sweetener and sugar-containing soda and risk of lymphoma and leukemia in men and women
- http://ajcn.nutrition.org/content/96/6/1419.abstract?ijkey= 06d1a2869308b45e73afc6559563b8f83fafa0bd&keytype2= tf_ipsecsha

- Neotame: Is this more-dangerous-than-aspartame sweetener hiding in your food? http://articles.mercola.com/sites/articles/ archive/2012/03/28/neotame-more-toxic-than-aspartame. aspx

Cereal grains

- Percy Schmeiser http://www.monsanto.com/newsviews/pages/percy-schmeiser.aspx

- Monsanto Canada Inc. vs. Schmeiser https://en.wikipedia.org/wiki/Monsanto_Canada_Inc_v_ Schmeiser

- Metals and arsenic in eye shadows. *Contact Dermatitis.* (2001) http://www.ncbi.nlm.nih.gov/pubmed/10644018

- Adoption of genetically engineered crops in the U.S. http://www.ers.usda.gov/data-products/adoption-of-genetically-engineered-crops-in-the-us/recent-trends-in-ge-adoption.aspx

- Developmental fluoride neurotoxicity: A systematic review and meta-analysis. (2012) http://www.ncbi.nlm.nih.gov/pubmed/22820538

Daily use items to avoid

- Analysis of plasticiser migration to meat roasted in plastic bags by SPME-GC/MS
  http://www.ncbi.nlm.nih.gov/pubmed/25704701

CHAPTER 15: THE NEW DEAL FOR DIABETICS

- Type 1 diabetes and prolonged fasting
  http://www.ncbi.nlm.nih.gov/pubmed/17367310

CHAPTER 16: EATING REAL

- Lethal algae take over beaches in northern France
  http://www.theguardian.com/world/2009/aug/10/france-brittany-coast-seaweed-algae

- Court rules France responsible in toxic algae case
  http://www.dailymail.co.uk/wires/ap/article-2701172/Court-rules-France-responsible-toxic-algae-case.html

- McDonald's burger looks the same – 14 years later. Time.com.
  http://newsfeed.time.com/2013/04/25/mcdonalds-burger-looks-the-same-14-years-later/

Water

- Total and specific fluid consumption as determinants of bladder cancer risk
  http://onlinelibrary.wiley.com/doi/10.1002/ijc.21587/abstract

- Over 300 pollutants in U.S. tap water
  http://www.ewg.org/tap-water

- Centers for Disease Control and Prevention – 2012 CDC Water Fluoridation Statistics
  http://www.cdc.gov/fluoridation/statistics/2012stats.htm

Meat

- Why processed meat is bad for you
  http://authoritynutrition.com/why-processed-meat-is-bad

- Hogging it; estimates of antimicrobial abuse in livestock
  http://www.iatp.org/files/Hogging_It_Estimates_of_
  Antimicrobial_Abuse_in.pdf

Poultry

- Chicken more popular than beef in U.S. for first time in 100 years
  http://www.huffingtonpost.com/2014/01/02/chicken-vs-beef_n_4525366.html

- Arsenic-based animal drugs and poultry
  http://www.fda.gov/AnimalVeterinary/SafetyHealth/
  ProductSafetyInformation/ucm257540.htm

- Summary Report of Poultry Imports Report for December 2015
  http://www.sapoultry.co.za/pdf-statistics/summary-imports-report.pdf

- Bovine Somatotropin (BST)
  http://www.fda.gov/AnimalVeterinary/SafetyHealth/
  ProductSafetyInformation/ucm055435.htm

Fish

- Farm-raised salmon poisoned with petrochemicals
  http://www.naturalhealth365.com/0890_farm_raised_
  salmon.html/

- Seafood selector
  http://seafood.edf.org

Sugar and fructose

- Uric acid and hypertension: Cause or effect? (2010)
  http://www.ncbi.nlm.nih.gov/pubmed/20425019

- Pediatric nonalcoholic fatty liver disease
  http://contemporarypediatrics.modernmedicine.com/
  contemporary-pediatrics/content/tags/biomarker/
  pediatric-nonalcoholic-fatty-liver-disease

- Consumption of honey, sucrose, and high-fructose corn
  syrup produces similar metabolic effects in glucose-tolerant
  and -intolerant individuals
  http://jn.nutrition.org/content/early/2015/09/02/
  jn.115.218016.abstract

Sweeteners

- Sugar substitutes – what's safe and what's not
  http://articles.mercola.com/sites/articles/
  archive/2013/10/07/sugar-substitutes.aspx

- Consumption of artificial sweetener and sugar-containing
  soda and risk of lymphoma and leukemia in men and
  women

- http://ajcn.nutrition.org/content/96/6/1419.abstract?ijkey=
  06d1a2869308b45e73afc6559563b8f83fafa0bd&keytype2=
  tf_ipsecsha

- Neotame: Is this more-dangerous-than-aspartame
  sweetener hiding in your food?
  http://articles.mercola.com/sites/articles/
  archive/2012/03/28/neotame-more-toxic-than-aspartame.
  aspx

Cereal grains

- Percy Schmeiser
  http://www.monsanto.com/newsviews/pages/percy-
  schmeiser.aspx

- Monsanto Canada Inc. vs. Schmeiser
  https://en.wikipedia.org/wiki/Monsanto_Canada_Inc_v_
  Schmeiser

- Metals and arsenic in eye shadows. *Contact Dermatitis.*
  (2001)
  http://www.ncbi.nlm.nih.gov/pubmed/10644018

- Adoption of genetically engineered crops in the U.S.
  http://www.ers.usda.gov/data-products/adoption-of-
  genetically-engineered-crops-in-the-us/recent-trends-in-
  ge-adoption.aspx

- Developmental fluoride neurotoxicity: A systematic review
  and meta-analysis. (2012)
  http://www.ncbi.nlm.nih.gov/pubmed/22820538

Daily use items to avoid

- Analysis of plasticiser migration to meat roasted in plastic bags by SPME-GC/MS
  http://www.ncbi.nlm.nih.gov/pubmed/25704701

CHAPTER 17: GUT HEALTH

- Surface area of the digestive tract – revisited. *Scandinavian Journal of Gastroenterology*
  http://informahealthcare.com/doi/abs/10.3109/00365521.2014.898326

- Isotropic fractionator: A simple, rapid method for the quantification of total cell and neuron numbers in the brain
  http://www.jneurosci.org/content/25/10/2518.full

- Vagus nerve stimulation in chronic treatment-resistant depression: Preliminary findings of an open-label study
  http://bjp.rcpsych.org/content/189/3/282.full

- That gut feeling. American Psychological Association.
  http://www.apa.org/monitor/2012/09/gut-feeling.aspx

- The scientific basis for probiotic strains of lactobacillus.
  http://aem.asm.org/content/65/9/3763

CHAPTER 18: WHAT BANTING FORGOT: MIND AND MOVEMENT

- New York City Marathon: Finisher demographics
  http://www.tcsnycmarathon.org/about-the-race/results/finisher-demographics

- Fauja Singh
  https://en.wikipedia.org/wiki/Fauja_Singh

CHAPTER 19: MIND MANAGEMENT: STRESS & SLEEP

- Franklin, B. *The Autobiography of Benjamin Franklin*.

- A sleep epidemic. Czeisler, C. Tedx Cambridge
  http://j.mp/1Cc9NXR

- Sleep and use of electronic devices in adolescence: Results from a large population-based study.
  http://j.mp/1N1neeP

- Suppression of melatonin secretion in some blind patients by exposure to bright light.
  http://www.ncbi.nlm.nih.gov/pubmed/7990870

- Dark chocolate intake buffers stress reactivity in humans. Wirtz P.H., von Känel R., Meister R.E., et al.

- Nocturnal awakenings and comorbid disorders in the American general population. (2006)
  http://j.mp/1MWgcd4

CHAPTER 20: MOVE

- A prospective study of cardiorespiratory fitness and breast cancer mortality.
  http://www.ncbi.nlm.nih.gov/pubmed/19276861

- Epidemiology of sedentary behaviour in office workers.
  http://phirn.org.uk/files/2013/01/SClemes-Epidemiology-of-sedentarybehaviour-in-office-workers.pdf

- Effects of interval walking on physical fitness in middle-aged individuals.
  http://www.ncbi.nlm.nih.gov/pubmed/23804371

CHAPTER 21: BODY BALANCE

- Falls among older adults: an overview.
  http://www.cdc.gov/HomeandRecreationalSafety/Falls/
  adultfalls.html

CHAPTER 22: GROWING MUSCLE LEGALLY

- How the sauna affects the endocrine system.
  http://www.ncbi.nlm.nih.gov/pubmed/3218898

- Are saunas the next big performance-enhancing "drug"?
  http://articles.mercola.com/sites/articles/
  archive/2014/05/24/sauna-benefits.aspx

CHAPTER 23: YOU LIE! EAT LESS, EXERCISE MORE

- Effects of dieting and exercise on resting metabolic rate and
  implications for weight management
  http://fampra.oxfordjournals.org/content/16/2/196.full

- 'Ambulance drone' could drastically increase heart attack
  survival
  http://www.iflscience.com/health-and-medicine/
  ambulance-drone-could-drastically-increase-heart-attack-
  survival

- Estimated calorie needs per day by age, gender, and
  physical activity level.
  http://www.cnpp.usda.gov/sites/default/files/usda_food_
  patterns/EstimatedCalorieNeedsPerDayTable.pdf

- *The American Meal* by Dr Winston Craig

FURTHER READING

In addition to trawling through hundreds of medical journal articles, here are some of the books I read while (or before) writing this book.

Ancestral
- *Before the dawn: Recovering the lost history of our ancestors* by Nicholas Wade
- *Sapiens* by Yuval Noah Harari
- *The third chimpanzee* by Jared Diamond

Balance
- *Better balance: Easy exercises to improve stability and prevent falls* by Suzanne E. Salamon & Bradley D. Manor
- *Whole body barefoot* by Katy Bowman

Diet and health
- *Good calories, bad calories: Fats, carbs, and the controversial science of diet and health* by Gary Tuabes
- *The diet delusion* by Gary Taubes
- *The hormone cure* by Sara Gottfried
- *The real meal revolution: The radical, sustainable approach to healthy eating* by Tim Noakes, Jonno Proudfoot and Sally-Ann Creed
- *Low carb diet strategies you don't know about* by Susan Campbell
- *The warrior diet* by Ori Hofmeckler

Paleo/Primal

- *The primal connection* by Mark Sisson
- *The paleo approach* by Sarah Ballantyne
- *The paleo diet for athletes* by Loren Cordain and Joe Friel
- *Primal body, primal mind* by Nora T. Gedgaudas

Other

- *The art and science of low carbohydrate performance* by Jeff Volek and Stephen Phinney
- *The science of leaky gut syndrome* by Case Adams
- *Sweat therapy* by Stephen A. Colmant
- *An introduction to coping with low self-esteem* by Melanie Fennell and Lee Brosan

Videos

Here are a few interesting videos to watch:

- Why exercise really is the best medicine by Professor Daniel Lieberman
  http://j.mp/1WQboKn
- Survival of the fleetest, smartest, or fattest? Human evolution 150 years after Darwin by Professor Daniel Lieberman
  http://j.mp/1TF2a4d
- The aetiology of obesity Part 1 of 6: A new hope by Jason Fung
  http://j.mp/1TJzOHo
- The two big lies of type 2 diabetes by Dr Jason Fung
  http://j.mp/1RuSU0E
- Why fasting bolsters brain power: Mark Mattson at TEDx Johns Hopkins University
  http://j.mp/1LTWpcq

- The world according to Monsanto
  http://j.mp/1RuT3Ru
- IGF-1 Insulin-like Growth Factor by Professor Luigi Fontana
  http://j.mp/1n40mF4
- Sugar: The bitter truth by Professor Robert Lustig
  http://j.mp/1TF2Y98
- 7 ways to rock cortisol & manage your stress by Dr. Sara
  Gottfried
  http://j.mp/1UqfiLg
- Dr. Mercola & Dr. Greger on How not to die
  http://j.mp/21plVTq
- King Corn – Documentary about two friends, one acre of
  corn, and the subsidized crop that drives America
  http://j.mp/1LkKsS6
- The deeper roots of health and diet as told by our ancestor's
  ancestors by Dr Ron Rosedale
  http://j.mp/1oOlVLu
- A sleep epidemic by Professor Charles Czeisler
  (TEDxCambridge 2011)
  http://j.mp/1oFPnTq

THE FOOD INSULIN INDEX

Food	FII	GI
With permission: The University of Sydney *School of Life and Environmental Sciences and Charles Perkins Centre* *Professor Jennie Brand-Miller*		
Note: Some examples of low GI foods with high insulin responses are bolded for reference. Protein with high branch chain amino acid content evokes larger than expected insulin responses.		
	Food Insulin Index	Glycaemic Index
Glucose (Glucodin Energy Powder)	100	100
Dairy Products		
Cream cheese (Coles)	**18**	**0**
93% Fat-free cheddar cheese (Dairy Farmers)	**20**	**0**
Full cream milk (Dairy Farmers)	24	31
Cheddar cheese (Coles)	**33**	**0**
1% Fat milk (Dairy Farmers)	34	29
Reduced-fat cottage cheese (Dairy Farmers)	**40**	**10**
Low-fat processed cheese slice (Kraft Foods Ltd)	**42**	**10**
Low-fat cottage cheese (Bulla Dairy Foods)	**52**	**10**
Skim milk (Dairy Farmers)	60	29
Peach-mango frozen yoghurt (Streets Blue Ribbon)	64	51
Vanilla ice-cream (Dairy Bell)	65	50
Low-fat vanilla ice-cream (Coles)	69	43

Low-fat strawberry yoghurt (Dairy Farmers)	84	31
Breads, Cereals, Grains, Rice & Pasta		
All-Bran Original (Kellogg's Foods Inc, Australia)	23	30
Porridge (Uncle Toby's Inc, Australia)	29	57
White pasta, spirals, boiled (San Remo)	29	46
Wholemeal pasta, boiled (San Remo)	29	42
Tortilla, white, corn (San Diego Tortilla Factory, Australia)	36	49
100% Natural Granola Oats, Honey & Raisins (Quaker Oats Inc, USA)	41	44
Grain bread (Tiptop Bakeries Inc)	41	50
Lentils in tomato sauce (Australia)	42	37
Brown rice, boiled (Ricegrowers Inc)	45	72
Special K (Kellogg's Foods Inc, Australia)	48	54
Cracklin' Oat Bran (Kellogg Foods Inc, USA)	48	55
Honeysmacks (Kellogg Foods Inc. Australia)	49	71
Soy-Lin grain bread (Burgen)	52	36
Sustain (Kellogg Foods Inc, Australia)	52	55
Cornflakes (Kellogg Foods Inc. Australia)	55	77
All-Bran Complete Wheat Flakes (Kellogg's Foods Inc, USA)	55	60
Great Grains (Kraft Foods Inc, USA)	57	74
7 Wholegrain Puffs (Kashi)	59	65
Honey Bunches of Oats (Post Foods Inc, USA)	61	63
Cheerios (General Mills Inc)	63	74
Lucky Charms (General Mills Inc)	69	69
Raisin bran (Kellogg's Foods Inc, USA)	69	61
Wholemeal bread (Riga Bakeries, Australia)	70	74
Frosted Flakes (Kellogg Foods Inc, USA)	72	55
White bread (Sunblest, Tiptop Pty Ltd)	73	70

Wheaties (General Mills Inc)	78	75
Cornflakes (Kellogg Foods Inc, USA)	82	81
Special K (Kellogg's Foods Inc, USA)	86	69
Original Shredded Wheat (Post Foods Inc, USA)	91	75
Rice Bubbles (Kellogg Foods Inc, Australia)	94	88
Grapenuts (Post Foods Inc, USA)	110	75
Fruit & Fruit Juice		
Avocado, raw, peeled (USA)	4	0
Seedless raisins (Sunbeam Food Inc ,Australia)	31	64
Red Delicious apple, raw (Australia)	43	36
Orange, raw, peeled (Australia)	44	42
Apple juice (Berrivale, Australia)	47	39
Peaches canned in juice (SPC Ardmona, Australia)	54	40
Orange juice (Mr Juicy, Australia)	55	53
Banana, raw, peeled (Australia)	59	52
Black grapes, raw (Australia)	60	50
Peaches canned in syrup (SPC Ardmona, Australia)	65	58
Honeydew melon, raw (Australia)	93	62
Vegetables & Legumes		
Coleslaw (Coles)	20	39
Canned navy beans (Eden Organic, USA)	23	31
Frozen corn (McCain Foods Pty Ltd)	39	47
Carrot juice, fresh (Australia)	41	43
Tomato pasta Sauce (Paul Newman)	41	31
Baked beans (Franklins)	**88**	**44**
Potato, russet, peeled and boiled (Australia)	88	78
Meat & Protein Alternatives		
Walnuts (Lucky California)	5	0
Short-cut bacon (Primo Smallgoods)	9	0

Bologna (Australia)	11	0
Peanut butter (Kraft Foods Inc, Australia)	11	14
Peanuts, salted and roasted (Grocery Wholesalers Inc, Australia)	15	14
Frankfurter/hot dog (Australia)	16	28
Tuna in oil, drained (Coles)	16	0
Roast chicken, without skin (Woolworth Inc)	**17**	**0**
Chicken, pan-fried with skin (Australia)	**19**	**0**
Prawns, boiled and peeled (Findus Seafood Deli)	**21**	**0**
Tofu (Soyco)	21	15
Eggs, poached (Australia)	**23**	**0**
Beef taco (Bruce Foods Corporation, USA)	24	39
Tuna in water, drained (Coles)	**26**	**0**
Beef steak, grilled (Australia)	**37**	**0**
White fish (Ling) fillet (Australia)	**43**	**0**
Battered fish fillet (Coles)	54	38
Fats & Oils		
Butter (Western Star Original)	2	0
Olive oil (Australia)	3	0
Beverages		
Gin, 40% alcohol (Australia)	1	0
White wine, 11% alcohol (Australia)	3	0
Beer, 4.9% alcohol (Budweiser, Australia)	20	66
Coca-Cola (Coca-Cola Amatil Inc)	44	53
Ice tea (Narkena Ltd)	69	59
Orange-mango fruit drink (Frosts Food & Beverage, Singapore)	76	67
Confectionery		
Milk chocolate (Hershey Foods Inc, USA)	34	43
Snickers bar (Masterfoods, USA)	37	42

Sherbet (Nestle Pty Ltd, Australia)	76	59
Mars bar (Mars Confectionary Inc, Australia)	89	62
Jellybeans (Grocery Wholesalers Inc. Australia)	117	78
Snacks		
Chocolate chip cookie (Chips Ahoy)	33	50
Muesli bar (Uncle Toby's Inc)	34	56
Honey-raisin bran muffin (Sun Maid, USA)	37	56
Popcorn (Uncle Toby's Inc)	39	66
Cinnamon swirl pastry (Bimbo Bakeries, USA)	42	40
Corn chips (The Smith's Snackfood)	45	42
Jatz cracker (Arnotts, Australia)	45	55
Potato chips (The Smith's Snackfood)	45	60
Apple pie (Sara Lee)	47	41
Reduced-fat chocolate chip cookie (Chips Ahoy, USA)	49	50
40% Reduced-fat potato chips (Cape Cod Potato Chip Company)	51	60
Super moist yellow cake with chocolate frosting (Betty Crocker, USA)	53	42
Donut with cinnamon sugar (Woolworths)	54	76
Fat-free oatmeal raisin cookie (Archway Cookies Inc)	54	54
Croissant (Woolworths)	58	67
Panjacks (White Wings Pty Ltd)	58	67
Chocolate brownie with frosting (White Wings)	60	38
Raspberry jam (Cottees)	62	51
Water crackers (Grocery Wholesalers)	64	78
Chocolate chip cookies (Arnotts Biscuits Ltd, Australia)	67	62

Blueberry streusel muffin (Pinnacle Foods Group LLC, USA)	69	55
Fat-free blueberry muffin (Continental Mills Pty Ltd)	69	71
97% Fat-free pretzels (Parkers)	74	84
Original Pancake & Waffle Mix (Quaker Oats)	110	67
Mixed meals & take-away foods		
Beef lasagne (Sara Lee Bakery Pty Ltd)	34	38
Cheese pizza (McCains, Australia)	47	60
French fries (McCain's Foods Inc)	54	70
French fries (McDonald's Inc)	57	70

Printed in Great Britain
by Amazon